Childhood Antecedents of Multiple Personality

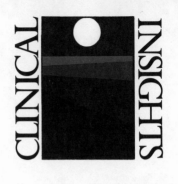

Childhood Antecedents of Multiple Personality

**Edited by
Richard P. Kluft, M.D., Ph.D.**

*Assistant Clinical Professor of Psychiatry,
Temple University School of Medicine; and
Attending Psychiatrist,
The Institute of the Pennsylvania Hospital*

AMERICAN PSYCHIATRIC PRESS, INC.
Washington, D.C.

© 1985 American Psychiatric Association

Manufactured in the U.S.A.

First printing--August 1985
Second printing--February 1987
Third printing--May 1988
Fourth printing--April 1989

The paper used in this publication meets the minimum requirements of American National Standard for Information Sciences—Permanence of Paper for Printed Library Materials, ANSI Z39.48-1984. ∞™

Library of Congress Cataloging in Publication Data

Main entry under title:

Childhood antecedents of multiple personality.

(Clinical insights)
Partly based on a symposium, "Aspects of Multiple Personality in Childhood," held during the 137th Annual Meeting of the American Psychiatric Association, 1984, in Los Angeles, Calif.
Includes bibliographies.
1. Multiple personality in children—Congresses. 2. Multiple personality in children—Etiology—Congresses. 3. Child abuse—Congresses. I. Kluft, Richard P., 1943-   . II. American Psychiatric Association, Meeting (137th:1984:Los Angeles, Calif.). III. Series. [DNLM: 1. Mental Disorders—in infancy & childhood—congresses. 2. Multiple-Personality Disorder—etiology—congresses. WM 173.6 C536]
RJ506.M84C48   1985   616.85′236   85-5986
ISBN 0-88048-082-3 (pbk.)

Contents

Contributors

BENNETT G. BRAUN, M.D., M.S.
Instructor, Department of Psychiatry, Rush Medical College;
and Clinical Associate Professor, Department of Psychology,
University of Illinois, Chicago

PHILIP M. COONS, M.D.
Assistant Professor of Psychiatry, Indiana University School of Medicine;
and Staff Psychiatrist, Larue D. Carter Memorial Hospital,
Indianapolis

EDWARD J. FRISCHHOLZ, M.A.
Department of Psychology and Office of Applied Psychological Services,
University of Illinois, Chicago

JEAN GOODWIN, M.D., M.P.H.
Director of Joint Programs, Milwaukee County Mental Health Program;
and Medical College of Wisconsin, Milwaukee

RICHARD E. HICKS, M.D.
Associate Professor, Department of Mental Health Sciences,
Hahnemann University Medical School; and Director of Education and
Training, Friends Hospital, Philadelphia

RICHARD P. KLUFT, M.D., Ph.D.
Assistant Clinical Professor of Psychiatry,
Temple University School of Medicine; and Attending Psychiatrist,
The Institute of the Pennsylvania Hospital, Philadelphia

FRANK W. PUTNAM, JR., M.D.
Neuropsychiatry Branch, National Institute of Mental Health,
Bethesda, Maryland

ROBERTA G. SACHS, Ph.D.
Private practice, Highland Park, Illinois

CORNELIA B. WILBUR, M.D.
Professor Emeritus, Department of Psychiatry,
University of Kentucky College of Medicine, Lexington

Introduction: Multiple Personality Disorder in the 1980s

A rapidly growing body of recent clinical and research contributions has substantially advanced our understanding of multiple personality disorder. As a consequence, this condition is gradually emerging from the shadowy realm of those psychiatric rarities, obscurities, and curiosities long surrounded by fascination, controversy, and skepticism. Multiple personality disorder is beginning to take its place among the recognized mental disorders. Although it is premature to consider this transition accomplished, and naive to assume the process will be completed without certain vicissitudes, considerable progress has been made in a rather brief period of time.

Greaves (1) noted that the 19th and 20th century clinical literature on multiple personality disorder was dominated by single case studies. Before 1980, the only large series of multiple personality disorder cases reported in the literature was that of Allison (2). In short order, Bliss (3), Braun (4), Kluft (5, 6), and Putnam et al. (7) described series of between 14 and 171 cases. It is well known that a number of experienced clinicians have not yet published their own comparable series. In his foreword to a *Psychiatric Clinics of North America* special 1984 issue on multiple personality disorder, Braun reported knowing of "approximately 1,000 cases" then in treatment with various therapists (8). My own poll of 70 mental health professionals who came as students to a recent course on multiple personality disorder revealed that they had encountered 267 such patients. Approximately 60 were currently treating individuals with multiple personality disorder. Clearly, the days of regarding multiple personality disorder as a rarity undeserving of scientific study are nearing an end.

As increasing numbers of multiple personality disorder patients are identified, it becomes possible to move toward correlating and researching psychopathological and psychophysiological phenomena that anecdotal reports can only describe, and that single case studies can only begin to document. Putnam has reviewed the history of 20th-century efforts to research multiple personality disorder (9). He has outlined both the models available for its exploration, and the practical considerations that influence subject selection and protocol design (10). It now is possible to begin to ask basic questions about multiple personality disorder and to evolve research strategies that may, in time, lead to reasonable answers.

The major findings of recently published explorations of multiple personality disorder can be summarized succinctly:

1. Multiple personality disorder is not rare (3–7). Its incidence is, however, unknown. The myth of rarity contributes to both its underdiagnosis and its misdiagnosis. In the series of 100 patients studied by National Institute of Mental Health (NIMH) workers, an average of 6.8 years had elapsed between these patients' first mental health assessments and their being diagnosed accurately (7, 11).

2. The psychophysiological and neurophysiological correlates of the separate personalities can be studied. They appear to hold up when measured against standard and real simulator controls. Nevertheless, investigators caution that in this area, as in any new field, first results must be regarded as preliminary. One must hedge tentative interpretations of the data by acknowledging the possibility that some unanticipated confounding systematic artifact may yet be discovered that leads to a revision of our current understandings (9, 12–14).

3. This condition is highly correlated with traumatic experiences during childhood. These usually, but not inevitably, involve child abuse (7, 15; Chapters 1–9 of this monograph).
4. This condition is highly responsive to psychotherapy (6).
5. Stable unification of the personality is achievable and has been documented by a follow-up study (6).
6. Commonly expressed concerns over risks of iatrogenesis and artifactual augmentation of the condition appear to have been greatly overemphasized. Working with the separate personalities does not reinforce them, nor does it worsen pathology. This may appear to be the case early in treatment; but, in fact, such an approach paves the way for their eventual mutual identification, empathy, and unification (6, 7, 16–19).
7. Individuals who develop multiple personality disorder are dissociation-prone (6). Recent studies support this long-standing clinical impression by demonstrating that multiple personality disorder patients are highly hypnotizable (20). They respond well to a variety of hypnotherapeutic interventions (5).
8. The circumspect and judicious use of hypnosis in the therapy of multiple personality disorder is benign and constructive. Previously expressed cautions appear to have been overstated. Misadventure can follow the misuse of hypnosis, as it would the misuse of any modality (5, 6, 17, 19).

Workers in the field have long been struck by the unfortunate impact of multiple personality disorder upon its victims. While some multiple personality disorder patients function adequately or even exceptionally, many are more or less incapacitated. All suffer. The cost and loss to the afflicted individuals, their loved ones, and society is immense. The "intriguing" and "fascinating" phenomena may capture the attention of the curious, the neophyte, and the dilettante. The difficulties involved in conceptualizing and explaining multiple personality disorder may stimulate the scientist and theoretician. But it is the stark misery of these patients and the ordeals they have endured that concern the experienced clinician.

An appreciation of this condition's potentially devastating impact and an awareness of its treatability combine to make the exploration of its childhood antecedents and manifestations timely, urgent, and of great potential importance. Recent advances and progress in the diagnosis, treatment, and exploration of adult multiple personality disorder suggest that its identification and treatment in childhood is desirable. The first reports of multiple personality disorder in childhood show that what is desirable is also eminently feasible (21).

Aspects of Multiple Personality in Childhood, the symposium that gave rise to this monograph, was presented at the 137th Annual Meeting of the American Psychiatric Association in Los Angeles. This symposium was the first ever organized to discuss multiple personality in childhood and to explore its antecedent causes. It was a coming together of clinicians and researchers to share current knowledge and establish a data base as a foundation for future work in this area. The original symposium's contributions have been augmented by additional studies, published for the first time in this monograph.

In Chapter 1, Dr. Jean Goodwin addresses a fundamental problem confronting anyone who works with those who say they have been abused—the problem of credibility. She offers an incisive and trenchant analysis of the pressures within individuals, professions, and societies to disavow the reality of what is too intolerable to accept.

In Chapter 2, Dr. Cornelia Wilbur draws upon her extensive experience with traumatized individuals in exploring the impact of child abuse upon a youngster's development, with particular reference to the creation of multiple personality disorder. She outlines the varieties of abuses encountered in the histories of such patients, and shares a number of clinical vignettes.

In Chapter 3, Drs. Bennett Braun and Roberta Sachs explicate a theory for the development of multiple personality disorder. They explore its predisposing, precipitating, and perpetuating factors, and propose that dissociation and severe distress are the essential preconditions of the disorder. They present a model for understanding the condition's etiology and apply the model to two case examples.

In Chapter 4, Dr. Frank Putnam places multiple personality disorder in the overall context of the dissociative disorders. He shows the association between this class of diagnostic entities and traumatic events. In a comprehensive review of the literature, he establishes that the connection between multiple personality disorder and overwhelming experiences is not an isolated correlation. In fact, dissociations of many varieties are similarly connected. The major differences seem to relate to the age of the victim at the time of the traumatization, and the nature of the traumata endured.

Edward Frischholz continues the exploration of connections between dissociation and child abuse in Chapter 5, by relating these topics to hypnosis and hypnotizability. He makes it possible to appreciate the importance of the literature of hypnosis to the study of multiple personality disorder. His work draws together a number of themes from previous chapters, and anticipates my comments on treatment in Chapter 8.

In Chapter 6, Dr. Bennett Braun describes his findings among the families of 18 patients suffering multiple personality disorder. His discovery that these patients' families include a large number of individuals who suffer dissociative disorders, including multiple personality disorder, offers powerful evidence for the transgenerational incidence of these conditions.

Closely related is Dr. Philip Coons's study, comparing children of 20 multiple personality disorder patients to children of 20 control cases, in Chapter 7. Dr. Coons documents a higher incidence of psychopathology among the children of the multiple personality disorder patients. He also finds a transgenerational incidence of multiple personality disorder, including a case of childhood multiple personality disorder.

In Chapter 8, I describe the evolution of a predictor instrument for childhood multiple personality disorder and its clinical validation on five actual cases of multiple personality disorder in children. I also discuss the presentations of the first cases of multiple personality disorder in children reported since 1840, draw distinctions between the adult and childhood forms of the condition, and offer comments on the treatment of the childhood form.

In Chapter 9, I present information on childhood cases, adult cases, and previously unpublished data on multiple personality disorder in older adults, in an attempt to describe the natural history and "life cycle" of multiple personality disorder. Data from childhood cases illuminate many of the most vexing dilemmas that continue to confound the accurate recognition of this diagnostic entity.

This monograph comes to a close with Dr. Richard E. Hicks's discussion of the preceding chapters, and his commentary on their implications for clinical practice and research.

Richard P. Kluft, M.D., Ph.D.

References

1. Greaves GB: Multiple personality: 165 years after Mary Reynolds. J Nerv Ment Dis 168:577-596, 1980

2. Allison RB: A new treatment approach for multiple personalities. Am J Clin Hypn 17:15-32, 1974

3. Bliss EL: Multiple personalities: a report of 14 cases with implications for schizophrenia and hysteria. Arch Gen Psychiatry 37:1388-1397, 1980

4. Braun BG: Hypnosis for multiple personalities, in Hypnosis in Clinical Medicine. Edited by Wain HJ. Chicago, Year Book Medical Publishers, 1980

5. Kluft RP: Varieties of hypnotic interventions in the treatment of multiple personality. Am J Clin Hypn 24:230-240, 1982

6. Kluft RP: Treatment of multiple personality. Psychiatr Clin North Am 7:9-29, 1984

7. Putnam FW, Post RM, Guroff JJ, et al: 100 cases of multiple personality disorder. Presented at the Annual Meeting of the American Psychiatric Association, New Research Abstract #77, New York, 1983

8. Braun BG: Foreword. Psychiatr Clin North Am 7:1-2, 1984

9. Putnam FW: The psychophysiologic investigation of multiple personality disorder: a review. Psychiatr Clin North Am 7:31-39, 1984

10. Putnam FW: The study of multiple personality disorder: general strategies and practical considerations. Psychiatric Annals 14:58-61, 1984

11. Kluft RP: An introduction to multiple personality disorder. Psychiatric Annals 14:19-24, 1984

12. Braun BG: Neurophysiologic changes in multiple personality due to integration: a preliminary report. Am J Clin Hypn 26:84-92, 1983

13. Braun BG: Psychophysiologic phenomena in multiple personality and hypnosis. Am J Clin Hypn 26:124-137, 1983

14. Brende JO: The psychophysiologic manifestations of dissociation. Psychiatr Clin North Am 7:41-50, 1984

15. Wilbur CB: Multiple personality and child abuse: an overview. Psychiatr Clin North Am 7:3-7, 1984

16. Wilbur CB: Treatment of multiple personality. Psychiatric Annals 14:27-31, 1984

17. Braun BG: Uses of hypnosis with multiple personality. Psychiatric Annals 14:34-40, 1984

18. Caul D: Group and videotape techniques for multiple personality disorder. Psychiatric Annals 14:43-50, 1984

19. Braun BG: Hypnosis creates multiple personality: myth or reality. Int J Clin Exp Hypn 32:191-197, 1984

20. Bliss EL: Multiple personalities, related disorders, and hypnosis. Am J Clin Hypn 25:114-123, 1983

21. Kluft RP: Multiple personality in childhood. Psychiatr Clin North Am 7:121-134, 1984

1

Credibility Problems in Multiple Personality Disorder Patients and Abused Children

Jean Goodwin, M.D., M.P.H.

1

Credibility Problems in Multiple Personality Disorder Patients and Abused Children

"It takes two to speak truth—one to speak and another to hear."
(Henry David Thoreau, *A Week on the Concord and Merrimack Rivers*)

Recent research is identifying a growing number of factors linking the syndrome of multiple personality disorder to child abuse. Putnam et al. (1), in a survey of 100 multiple personality patients undergoing treatment, found that more than 90 percent of those studied had been abused during their early years. More cases of multiplicity are being identified, in which protective service records clearly document the chaotic and psychotic family situations that dominated these patients' childhoods (2). This chapter focuses on yet another parallel between multiplicity and child abuse—the incredulity that both inspire in physicians.

One need look back only as far as papers and textbooks published in the 1960s and 1970s to document this incredulity factor. Most present-day psychiatrists were confidently taught, and tried to believe just as confidently, that multiple personality did not occur, but might be mentioned at times by female patients who were malingering or attention-getting, or who had been persuaded that this was their diagnosis by clumsy or cunning hypnotists (3–5); and that intrafamilial childhood sexual abuse (incest) did not actually occur, but might be mentioned at times by female patients who mistook their oedipal longings and fantasies for realities (6).

The credibility problems in multiple personality epitomize the

2

difficulties faced by the abuse victim within the mental health care delivery system. In these cases, professionals are incredulous not only of the existence of the disorder and of the patient's narratives about extremely severe childhood abuse, but most physicians also have difficulty believing even the most commonplace, concrete, and prosaic of the patient's statements. This incredulity is created by the patient's own habits of concealment, adaptive for survival in a traumatic childhood, but terribly confusing when they operate outside of awareness in adulthood.

The following is an example: A multiple personality patient experienced increased agitation and ultimately overdosed during an exacerbation of her chronic pelvic pain. The psychiatric crisis nurses who interviewed her did not believe the patient was really upset or in pain, or that she had overdosed, but admitted her to a psychiatric hospital when blood levels of the sedative she had ingested were found to be elevated. Staff in the psychiatric hospital did not believe she had multiple personality. They diagnosed her as having a borderline personality disorder with a factitious syndrome. The gynecologist, who, after several years, had come to believe that the sadistic sexual abuse she described really had taken place, believed the patient was experiencing remembered pain (her father had repeatedly manipulated her cervix with an ice pick). However, ultrasound studies revealed multiple cysts on both ovaries, and the patient was scheduled for surgery. At this point, the anesthetist did not believe the patient when she said she was allergic to adhesive tape. As a consequence, the surgery, although it relieved her pelvic pain, left the patient with an uncomfortable and completely preventable rash.

Clinicians who have worked extensively with patients suffering from multiple personality disorder know that this vignette is excerpted from an almost endless series of disbeliefs and misunderstandings. What is remarkable in this pattern is its similarity to patterns of disbelief of accounts given by abused children in general, and of reports made by sexually abused children in particular. Since sadistic sexual abuse is among the most characteristic abuse patterns in the life histories of patients who develop multiple personality disorder, it is possible that the credibility problems in both groups of victims share and stem from common sources (7). If patients with multiple personalities can be understood as abused children in adult bodies (whose childhood traumata and responses to those traumatizations have been preserved through time by dissociation), their problems in being believed are likely to be similar to the problems encountered by children who attempt to tell their stories at an earlier point in their lives.

This chapter reviews the history of professional disbelief of abused children and the possible causes for this "credibility gap," as they relate both to the defensive styles of professionals and to the modes of expression typical of abused children. In the spirit of Thoreau's aphorism about truth-telling, I will be listing the obstacles that interfere with the child abuse victim's ability to speak his or her particular truth, and with the physician's capacity to hear it.

PROFESSIONAL INCREDULITY ABOUT CHILD ABUSE

Iwan Bloch, a contemporary of Sigmund Freud, stated,"Children's declarations before the law are, for the truly experienced knower of children . . . absolutely worthless and without significance; all the more insignificant and all the more hollow the more often the child repeats the declaration and the more determined he is to stick to his statements" (8).

Child abuse, although well described by the French forensic physician, Tardieu, in 1860 (9), was not "officially" discovered by physicians and psychiatrists until Henry Kempe and Brandt Steele made child abuse a public policy issue in the 1950s (10). Before this time, physicians found it easier to believe that infants who presented with multiple fractures, multiple bruises, and subdural hematoma exhibited a genetic syndrome, rather than consider the possibility that such injuries indicated that they might have been beaten (11). Cases in the contemporary literature still describe children whose complaints about beatings are disbelieved, and who later meet violent deaths after being returned to abusive parents (12).

Several reviews of deaths attributed to child abuse report that most children who are over six months old at the time of death had been previously referred for child protective services; often social workers had closed these cases with a note to the effect that they did not believe abuse to be a serious problem in the soon-to-be murderous families (13, 14). Many professionals continue to balk at laws that require the reporting of child abuse. For example, as recently as 1972, private pediatricians accounted for only eight of 2,300 child abuse reports in New York City (15). Despite evidence that half of psychiatric patients were abused in childhood, psychiatrists have yet to implement standard interview schedules that would make questioning in this area routine (16).

Childhood sexual abuse is the category of abuse with the longest and most fascinating history of disbelief. Victim credibility has been the central issue in such cases since the Inquisition (17). As he began working with female patients who reported childhood seductions, Sigmund Freud came to realize that 16th-century Inquisitors had been processing similar narratives. "Why are their confessions under torture so like the communications made by my patients in psychological treatment?" he wrote of the accused witches (18). The Inquisitors interpreted the sexual accusations of those they interrogated as evidence that the devil had assumed the guise of a male relative in order to consummate intercourse with the woman who was, therefore, obviously a witch (19). Freud ultimately came to believe that such complaints represented oedipal fantasies that had been disguised as memories of actual sexual contact with the father (8). Curiously, both interpretations focused on the complainant, highlighting her pathology and encouraging her to alter or to disavow her complaint, which now could be reformulated as consorting with the devil or failing to distinguish an oedipal fantasy from an incestuous reality. In both systems, the accused male relative might never be interviewed, and the female complainant's very account could be used to indict her perceptions of reality.

Freud's ultimate endorsement of incredulity as the appropriate scientific response to a child's sexual accusations was in conformity with the contemporary wisdom of his day, that children and hysterics were not to be believed. There are, in fact, many sound arguments in favor of using developmental sensitivity in interpreting the communications of children; for example, to return to the Inquisition, witch-hunting went most out of control in those jurisdictions that allowed children to testify (20). However, the incredulity that Freud championed goes beyond this. For example, Freud published several cases in which a patient's account of prior sexual abuse was corroborated by a co-victim, a witness, or by the adult participant (21). He never published a case of a corroborated false account of sexual abuse. Yet, Freud later expressed embarrassment at his "credulity" in having believed stories of sexual seduction in childhood (22).

His incredulity was the more defensible stance, regardless of the evidence. This was underlined for me recently when a psychoanalytic colleague staunchly refused to believe that sexual abuse existed in a family where three daughters, one granddaughter, and one grandson had complained, and where medical evidence was available. Medical evidence itself is often misinterpreted to support an incredulous stance. Although French physicians in the 1800s published clear data that sexual assaults on children often occurred repeatedly and over long periods of time without leaving physical signs, the absence of such signs was, until recently, taken as irrefutable evidence that the child was lying (23).

In 1885, Brouardel, a contemporary of Freud, wrote that of 100 complaints of sexual abuse, 60 to 80 are unfounded (8). It is an ironic curiosity that these figures are similar to those found currently among another group, the parents of sexually abused children. Even after a legal finding of sexual abuse, 20 percent to 50 percent of these parents persist in alleging that the child lied (24). However, recent figures from professionals estimate that less than five percent of accusations are unfounded, and if one considers only those cases in which the child has made a statement, the figure drops to under one percent (25–27).

Most false accusations of sexual abuse are made by adults. The credibility issue that has become prominent now in this area is whether one can believe the child who says sexual abuse did not occur. As many as one-third of children who have been sexually abused consider falsely retracting their complaints under pressure from distraught parents and incredulous professionals (28). Often, children are openly coerced into retracting their statements. They are confronted with threats of psychiatric hospitalization, exile from the family, or physical punishment if they persist in their complaints. There is, in addition, a more subtle pressure on the child to produce a version of reality that respected adults are willing to acknowledge, even if this must be constructed at the price of dissociation and amnesia. It is likely that in the past physicians mistook these false retractions for truth and, thereby, overestimated the incidence of false accusations. Once again, it is not a new discovery that children tend to lie to protect their parents. Tardieu, in his 1860 monograph, described a child who was kept locked in a chest, beaten regularly, and vaginally penetrated with a block of wood. She invented falls and accidents to explain her injuries (9). Still, historically, the tendency of physicians has been to be more credulous of children's retractions than of their complaints.

SELF-PROTECTIVE ASPECTS OF THE PHYSICIAN'S INCREDULITY

"It is more ignominious to mistrust our friends than to be deceived by them." (Rochefoucauld, *Maxims*)

In this section I will not consider those aspects of physician incredulity that are appropriate responses to the child's narration; these will be covered in the next section. Here, I will consider only those factors that interfere with a physician's ability to be credulous of a particular account, regardless of the child's narrative style or reality contact. These are the aspects of the physician's incredulity that are rooted in personal defenses against fear, guilt, and anger.

Incredulity can be understood as an intellectualized variant of derealization; and, like the dissociative defenses, incredulity is an effective way to gain distance from terrifying realities. Thus, physicians can be counted on to routinely disbelieve child abuse accounts that are simply too horrible to be accepted without threatening their emotional homeostasis. Stories that will be disbelieved include those involving genital mutilation, the placing of objects into the vaginal, anal, or urethral openings, incest with multiple family members, incest pregnancies, and the protracted tying down or locking up of children. By placing limits on what we believe, we maintain for ourselves a more sane and manageable world. An example will, perhaps, clarify this point. In treating a woman with multiple personality, many of her alternate personalities (alters) described witnessing her father rape and murder girls and women. I suggested that she report these emerging memories to the authorities. When the authorities reported that three rape–murders had occurred in the two years since her father had moved to a nearby small town, I realized, in a wave of panic, that I had hoped the patient was merely fantasizing; and that I had been unprepared to accept the horrors of her narrative as truth.

Incredulity functions, as well, to combat more subtle anxiety, allowing the physician to believe that the patient and family are not as ill as they seem. Just as we hope that the positive guaiac test will be an error, or that the shadow on the chest film is only an artifact, we try to find as benign a view as we can of an accusation of child abuse. Incredulity protects both the physician and the family from unpleasant realities, such as investigating the physical and psychological consequences to the child, inquiring about other victims, going to Court to protect the child, or making a commitment to the hundreds of hours of treatment that may be necessary (29). As Sgroi has said, "I know of no other clinical situation in which the intervenor's payoff for denial . . . equals or exceeds . . . the participant's" (30).

In these cases, if the therapist is in any empathic contact at all with either one of the parents or with the child, guilt is unavoidable. The parent who has failed to control impulses, the parent who cannot show tenderness or who has failed to protect, the child who believes she is experiencing something that no other child has endured—and then has broken the secret of that terrible something—all suffer intolerable guilt. Disbelief is a way of undoing this series of transgressions and freeing the physician from worries about his or her own (or his or her parents') lack of impulse control, inability to care or to protect, and memories of painful, secret experiences.

Incredulity also shields the physician from the powerful anger and rage in these families. Parents who are clinically or subclinically paranoid may respond to confrontation about abuse with tirades that are simultaneously so pitiably persecuted and grandiosely terrifying that the physician is driven to recant as surely as is the child victim (31). Also, the victim is angry and preoccupied with revenge fantasies. This anger may be expressed in such indirect ways (for example, in the victim's persistent experiencing of the physician as a monster, a sadist, a rapist, or a murderer) that the physician may not even recognize his or her own responsive indignation before this translates into incredulity, one of the few expressions of anger permitted to the physician. Since, as physicians, we are prohibited by law and custom from abandoning bona fide patients, we must redefine intolerable patients as nonpatients in order to escape from them (32). Thus, the redefining of the angry child abuse victim as unabused can be likened to the redefining of the intractable pain patient as being without pain, or to the redefining of the disappointed, disabled patient as malingering.

Finally, believing a child's report about a sadistic sexual assault leaves the physician vulnerable to a barrage of sexual feelings. How does one react to the six-year-old who lifts her skirt and invites the therapist to tickle her underwear? It is all too easy for the clinician to overlook the query about the safety of the relationship, the crucial question that is always embedded in the child's "seductiveness" (33), and to become convinced that repetitive behaviors or discussions about the prior sexual abuse are deliberately intended to sexually entice or stimulate (34). Patient seductiveness is the rationalization typically brought forward by therapists who have become sexually involved with patients who are adult incest victims, or who have multiple personality disorder (35). Such involvements are not rare, and are merely the most personally and professionally disastrous of a spectrum of readjustments in sexual feeling and thinking that can be triggered by entering the world of these patients. Among the lesser hazards to the physician are decreased sexual desire, orgasmic dysfunction, withdrawal from physical contact with one's own children, and intense discomfort with the current balance of power between men and women.

WHY CHILDREN ARE NOT CREDIBLE

> "If she be a witch, she will not be able to weep." (Malleus Maleficarum, in Kors and Peters, *Witchcraft in Europe, 1100-1700*)
> "Wiping hands during testimony is almost always a sign of lying." (Anonymous judge, in Slovenko, *Psychiatry and Law*)

Consistency, association of appropriate emotions, calm confidence in the credibility of a narration—these are some criteria for truthfulness mentioned in world folklore and in forensic psychiatry textbooks. What is not clear is whether any of these criteria apply at all to normal children or, much less, to children who have been traumatized, who are experiencing dissociative symptoms, or who have strong desires not to be believed because of loyalty to and identification with the aggressor (36).

Let us consider, first, the purely developmental issues (37). The child, prior to the development of operational thinking, will mix accounts of fantasy and accounts of actual events, and may express memories through sensorimotoric reenactments, play, or physical symptoms rather than words. In latency, the child is able to narrate better, but still may fail to meet credibility criteria because the prepubertal suppression of sexuality precludes "appropriate" emotional responses (that is, those responses experienced by adults); these include sexual interest, attraction, jealousy, or horror of rape. When a child of this age describes a rape without weeping, her "brazen poise," as it was once called, may be taken as a sign that she is not describing an actual event (38). Unfortunately, when the incest victim in adolescence does, at last, develop "appropriate" emotional reactions to sexuality, she may be perceived as still lacking credibility, now by virtue of being "seductive" or "manipulative." Time and again, one observes teenaged victims disclosing their incest experiences at the precise moment when they are least likely to be believed; for example, when they have been caught breaking a rule, or when they have become pregnant by a boyfriend. Although this pattern makes emotional sense in terms of the teenaged victim's disillusion with her parents and scorn of their authority, these crisis-related complaints can be misconstrued easily as opportunistic lies.

With traumatized children, credibility problems multiply. Lenore Terr, a child psychiatrist, interviewed 23 of the 26 grade school children involved in the 1976 Chowchilla, California, school bus kidnapping (39). These children had been held by their kidnappers for 27 hours. Three masked men blocked the road with a van, took over the school bus at gunpoint, drove the children around in vans for 11 hours, and then transferred the children to a buried truck-trailer, which they covered with earth. The children spent 16 hours buried there before two of the older boys dug them out and all the children escaped. Interviewed between five and 13 months after the incident, 14 of the 23 children had major perceptual and cognitive distortions about the incident. Five had distorted memories of the appearance of the kidnapper; six had formulated theories about a nonexistent fourth kidnapper still dangerously at large; and three hallucinated entire scenes. Inaccurate time sequencing occurred in the narratives of eight children. Distortions were experienced even by the adolescents on the bus. They were the ones most active in efforts to escape and organize their own rescue, and the impact of their experiences upon their perceptions must influence our expectations for Court testimony by traumatized children.

Traumatization can induce distortions. Despite these distortions, however, amnesia, repression, and suppression were notably absent from the children's accounts; it may be that this developmentally linked, unflinching completeness is part of what makes it so difficult for adult physicians to listen to children's narratives of pain (40). In addition, all children had symptoms of fear or anxiety; five children exhibited compulsive retelling of the story; six had elaborate aggressive revenge fantasies; and nine were in depressive states with regressive, dream-like behaviors. Any of these trauma-related symptoms might be used to question a child's credibility.

Trauma-related distortions multiply when a family member has traumatized the child, when this person has enlisted the child as an accomplice in a conspiracy of silence, and when a lifetime's experience has convinced the child that he or she is a second-class citizen without rights. The distorted narrative that emerges from these pressures in incest situations has been described by Roland Summit as the "accommodation syndrome" (41). The incest victim does not complain, sometimes for years; she does not tell her mother, run away, or call for help. When she does tell someone, she may do so in a partial or cryptic way, may insist on secrecy, or may pledge that if police are involved, she herself will disavow her story. She may be deeply cynical about the good intentions of those in authority. She will feel guilty about her disloyalty in betraying her parents, and often will appear guilty or uncertain to her examiners. Sacrificing truth for acceptance and stability may be a familiar way of life by the time incest is disclosed. As many as 20 percent of incest victims develop a pattern of conduct disorder that includes lying, as well as running away, school problems, and drug use (42). Those child abuse victims who develop the full sociopathic syndrome present credibility problems that may defy currently available psychotherapeutic approaches.

If, in addition to all of the above, this incest victim is able to persuade herself at moments that nothing really happened, she becomes incredible indeed. Partial memories and derealized memories are routine in incest victims; some feign sleep during the sexual contact, which is often initiated while the child is actually asleep. Even partial amnesia or mild dissociation can be associated with dream-like, stereotyped, affectless impersonal accounts, which vary with each retelling. The child's wish that the abuse not be happening (which triggered the initial dissociation) persists as a wish that her narration not be believed, so that both she and her parents can avoid facing their real relationship (43). If actual multiplicity is at issue, the victim's credibility is further impaired by her tendency to talk about herself in the third person (which may be associated with tendencies to refer to alters or imaginary playmates as if they were real others) and by the differing partial memories and screen memories that each personality has for a single event.

WHY PATIENTS WITH MULTIPLE PERSONALITY ARE NOT BELIEVED

"Fact or fiction—in the end you can't distinguish between them—you just have to choose." (Graham Greene, *Monsignor Quixote*)

What does this analysis of the problems that professionals experience in believing abused children tell us about multiple personalities?

First, it leads us to the hypothesis that patients with multiple personality disorder are the least credible of victims because they are among the most severely abused. The multiplicity of types of abuse, of perpetrators, and the bizarre sadistic details in their stories make doctors more horrified, more angry, and, therefore, more likely to defend by disbelieving. The more severely traumatized children are, the more likely they are to lie, to repeat woodenly, to hallucinate, to dissociate, to retract, and to not complain; they are, therefore, difficult to believe. Multiple personality patients who have experienced a lifetime of abuse at different developmental stages, and who have alters of various ages, display, in turn, the credibility problems associated with each developmental stage.

Second, we must ask how much the familial and professional disbelief of child abuse furthers the development of dissociative mechanisms in the child. A child with low self-esteem and great need for approval will manage her memories to suit the assertions of important adults. We have seen alter personalities emerge in one child when a parent disbelieved an abuse complaint. Part of the function of altering in personality, or otherwise repressing a traumatic event, is to make it easier for the child to participate in the family myth that nothing happened. When professionals join the family in insisting that nothing happened, these dissociative defenses are strengthened. Erik Erikson described the problem in

Freud's teenaged patient, Dora, as a crisis of fidelity that developed after her maritally unfaithful father abandoned her to be seduced by his friend (44). Erikson postulated that what such patients seek in a therapist is the capacity for fidelity. This implies more than credulity on the part of the therapist. It means a commitment to setting the historical record straight so that the patient's own identity and future can unfold; it means an absolute openness to the emotional truth of the patient as this emerges in associations, symptoms, transference, and, ultimately, in abreaction.

A third hypothesis generated from this review is that we observe, in interactions with patients with multiple personality disorder and abused children and their families, a shared negative hallucination. In medicine, we have given so little thought to this negative type of distortion that we do not even have a name for it. There is no named entity with which to contrast malingering and hysteria. To talk about "denial" of illness minimizes the extent of the reality distortion that occurs in these negative illusions. "Flight into health" conveys a more accurately eerie impression of the patient clambering onto a broom for a midnight flight. For example, pseudocyesis is a well defined hysterical symptom. But, until recently, very little had been written about its opposite; that is, about those women who remain oblivious of actual pregnancies until delivery, and who keep families and physicians in the dark, as well (45). In many ways, this last is the more remarkable phenomenon.

When we treat patients with multiple personality disorder, we discover that behind their well described hysterical conditions—the paralysis, the pain, the factitious fevers—there lie real conditions desperately camouflaged and cryptically expressed by the somatoform symptoms (46). This concealed reality almost always includes sadistic abuse in childhood. The multiple personality disorder patient and the physician cling to the series of false symptoms and false diagnoses in proportion to their mutual need to blot out the reality of the multiplicity, and to blot out the unbearable experiences of real pain that triggered it. Part of choosing to believe abused children and adult patients with multiple personality disorder is choosing to confront our own complicity in the wishing away of these unbearable childhood experiences (47, 48).

References

1. Putnam FW, Post RM, Guroff JJ, et al.: 100 cases of multiple personality disorder. Paper presented at the Annual Meeting of the American Psychiatric Association, New Research Abstract #77, New York, May, 1983

2. Kluft R: Multiple personality in childhood. Psychiatr Clin North Am 7:121-134, 1984

3. Kampman R: Hypnotically induced multiple personality: an experimental study. Int J Clin Exp Hypn 24:215-227, 1976

4. Leavitt HD: A case of hypnotically produced secondary and tertiary personalities. Psychoanal Rev 34:274-295, 1947

5. Harriman PL: A new approach to multiple personalities. Am J Orthopsychiatry 13:636-642, 1943

6. MacDonald JM: Rape: Offenders and Their Victims. Springfield, Il, Charles C Thomas, 1971

7. Saltman V, Solomon RS: Incest and the multiple personality. Psychol Rep 50:1127-1141, 1982

8. Masson JM: The Assault on Truth: Freud's Suppression of the Seduction Theory. New York, Farrar, Straus & Giroux, 1984

9. Tardieu A: Etude medio-legale sur les services et mauvais traitements exerces sur des enfants. Annales d'Hygiene Publique et de Medicine Legale 13:361-398, 1860

10. Kempe CH, Silverman FN, Steele BF, et al: The battered child syndrome. JAMA 181:17-24, 1962

11. Caffey J: Multiple fractures in long bones of infants suffering from chronic subdural hematomas. American Journal of Roentgenology 56:163-173, 1946

12. Elmer E: Children in Jeopardy: A Study of Abused Minors and Their Families. Pittsburgh, University of Pittsburgh Press, 1967

13. Goodwin J, Geil C: Why physicians should report child abuse: the example of sexual abuses, in Sexual Abuse: Incest Victims and Their Families. Boston, Wright/PSG, 1982

14. Scott PD: Fatal battered baby cases. Medicine, Science, and Law 13:197-206, 1973

15. Helfer RE: Why most physicians don't get involved in child abuse cases, and what to do about it. Children Today 4:28-32, 1975

16. Carmen EH, Rieber PP, Mills T: Victims of violence and psychiatric illness. Am J Psychiatry 141:378-383, 1984

17. Hilberman E: The Rape Victim. New York, Basic Books; and Washington, DC, The American Psychiatric Association, 1976

18. Freud S: The Origins of Psychoanalysis: Letters to Wilhelm Fliess. Drafts and Notes, 1887-1902. Edited by Bonaparte A, Freud A, Kris E. New York, Basic Books, 1954

19. Goodwin J: Cross-cultural perspectives on clinical problems of incest, in Sexual Abuse: Incest Victims and Their Families. Edited by Goodwin J. Boston, Wright/PSG, 1982

20. Monter EW: Witchcraft in France and Switzerland. Ithaca, NY, Cornell University Press, 1976

21. Balmary M: Psychoanalyzing Psychoanalysis. Baltimore, Johns Hopkins University Press, 1982

22. Freud S: An Autobiographical Study. Translated by Strachey J. London, Hogarth Press, 1935

23. Goodwin J, Willett A, Jackson R: Medical care for male and female incest victims and their parents, in Sexual Abuse: Incest Victims and Their Families. Edited by Goodwin J. Boston, Wright/PSG, 1982

24. Defrances V: Protecting the Child Victim of Sex Crimes Committed by Adults. Englewood, CO, American Humane Association, 1969

25. Goodwin J: Helping the child who reports incest: a case review, in Sexual Abuse: Incest Victims and Their Families. Edited by Goodwin J. Boston, Wright/PSG, 1982

26. Goodwin J, Sahd D, Rada R: Incest hoax: false accusations, false denials. Bull Am Acad Psychiatry Law 6:269-276, 1979

27. Cantwell HB: Sexual abuse of children in Denver, 1979: reviewed with implications for pediatric interventions and possible preventions. Child Abuse Negl 5:75-86, 1981

28. Nakashima I, Zakus GE: Incest: review and clinical experience. Pediatrics 60:696-701, 1977

29. Ounsted C, Oppenheimer R, Lindsay J: Aspects of bonding failure: the psychopathology and psychotherapeutic treatment of families of battered children. Dev Med Child Neurol 16:447-456, 1974

30. Sgroi S, Porter FS, Blick LC: Validation of Child Sexual Abuse, in Handbook of Clinical Intervention in Child Sexual Abuse. Lexington, MA, Lexington Books, 1982

31. Goodwin J: Persecution and grandiosity in incest fathers. Proceedings of the Seventh World Congress of Psychiatry (in press)

32. Goodwin J, Vogel A: Knowledge and use of placebo among house officers and nurses. Ann Intern Med 91:106-110, 1979

33. Krieger MJ, Rosenfeld AA, Gordon A, et al: Problems in the psychotherapy of children with a history of incest. Am J Psychother 34:81-88, 1980

34. De Young M: Case reports: the sexual exploitation of incest victims by helping professionals. Victimology 6:92-101, 1981

35. Watkins JG, Watkins H: Hazards to the therapist in the treatment of multiple personalities. Psychiatr Clin North Am 7:111-119, 1984

36. Rees K: The child's understanding of his past. Psychoanal Study Child 33:237-259, 1978

37. Goodwin J, Owen J: Incest from infancy to adulthood: a developmental approach to victims and families, in Sexual Abuse: Incest Victims and Their Families. Edited by Goodwin J. Boston: Wright/PSG, 1982

38. Bender L, Blau A: The reaction of children to sexual relations with adults. Am J Orthopsychiatry 7:500-518, 1937

39. Terr L: Children of Chowchilla: a study of psychic trauma. Psychoanal Study Child 34:552-623, 1979

40. Terr L: The child as witness, in Child Psychiatry and the Law. Edited by Schetky DH and Benedek EP. New York, Brunner/Mazel, 1980

41. Summit R: The child sexual abuse accommodation syndrome. Child Abuse Negl 7:177-193, 1983

42. Maisch H: Incest. New York, Stein and Day, 1972

43. Dickes R: The defensive function of an altered state of consciousness: a hypnoid state. J Am Psychoanal Assoc 13:356-403, 1965

44. Erikson E: Reality and actuality: an address. J Am Psychoanal Assoc 10:451-474, 1962

45. Silverblatt H, Goodwin J: Denial of pregnancy. Bulletin of Birth Psychology 4:13-25, 1983

46. Stoller R: Splitting: A Case of Feminine Masculinity. New York, International Psychoanalytic Library, 1974

47. Benedek E: The silent scream: countertransference reactions to victims. American Journal of Social Psychiatry 4:49-52, 1984

48. Miller A: For Your Own Good. New York, Farrar, Straus & Giroux, 1983

2

The Effect of Child Abuse on the Psyche

Cornelia B. Wilbur, M.D.

2

The Effect of Child Abuse
on the Psyche

Child abuse is a public health dilemma of epidemic proportions. A recent increase in public awareness and media attention to this ongoing and widespread human tragedy is welcome and long overdue. Whether this attention will lead us to come to grips with the tragedy of child abuse, however, remains to be seen. The subject of child abuse is extremely disturbing. We would like to believe that child abuse is infrequent and, when it occurs, that it happens in families most unlike our own.

In this chapter, I will not review the many reasons why it is difficult for people to accept the enormity of this problem, why they are inclined to disbelieve reports of its incidence and prevalence (which are invariably understatements: much abuse goes undetected and unreported), and why people often arrive, without conscious malice, at stances that ignore the overwhelming consequences of child abuse. Perhaps entire societies can suffer what Summit has called the "child abuse accommodation syndrome" (1) and erect defenses in order to accept a more congenial alternative reality (2). In Chapter 1 of this monograph, Dr. Jean Goodwin addressed one aspect of this failure to come to terms with the truth about child abuse: the incredulity of mental health professionals toward reports of abuse suffered by children. In this chapter, I will review the varied and often interrelated forms that child abuse may take, and examine the effects of these abuses upon the psyche.

TYPES OF ABUSE

The whole range of child abuse can be conceptualized as broad spectrums of non-nurturing (neglect, or harm by acts of omission) and active abuse (harm by acts of commission). Non-nurturing begins as an emotional neglect of the legitimate needs of the developing child, whether by intention, unavailability, or some form of deficit or incapacity in the caretaker. From this failure to appreciate and respond to the needs of the child, stems actual physical neglect. A child may not be held, comforted, bathed, kept warm, diapered, or fed adequately by a caretaker unable or unwilling to react to him or her empathetically and responsively. Non-nurturing often includes providing food that is inappropriate for an infant or child, or a diet that is inadequate in the basic substances that prevent vitamin and other deficiencies. The developmental lags and defects that result, of course, interact with and amplify the impacts of other forms of abuse.

Case Example 1

A patient was adopted by a childless couple. The wife immediately developed paranoid schizophrenia, and neglected the child's basic needs. The husband allowed his wife to remain at home and did not protect his daughter from the wife's bizarre and disturbed behaviors. The girl developed multiple personality disorder. During her successful treatment, she traced her roots and learned that while she was born out-of-wedlock and given up for adoption, her biological parents later married and had many children. She sought out and met her siblings. She found that while their appearances and temperaments were quite similar to her own, she was seven inches shorter than any other female member of the family. Her doctor believes she had suffered rickets and other avitaminoses as a child.

The other type of abuse, active abuse, includes sexual abuse. Even infants and very young children may be abused sexually, and such incidents are far from infrequent. In 1978, the Orange

County Mental Health Center, in Orange County, California, reported a 30 percent incidence of incest among the female patients who were admitted to the clinic for treatment. This is not an isolated phenomenon. As incest survivors' groups have proliferated, and increasing numbers of victims come forward to share their experiences, the full spectrum of this problem is beginning to emerge.

We would like to believe most sexual abuse of children is done by strangers (most often drifters and "perverts"), or occasionally by individuals who insinuate themselves into settings in which children are vulnerable and easily accessible (that is, schools, daycare centers, clubs, camps, and so forth). Certainly, such instances are readily called to the public's attention. Most sexual abuse, however, occurs within the family or the neighborhood. Both male and female infants and youngsters may be sexually abused by both parents and other relatives of both sexes. Female children have been subject both to rape and to other forms of abuse as sexual objects by their fathers, brothers, male neighbors, or the paramours of their mothers, sisters, or other caretakers. Male children can be abused by comparable female figures. Of course, the homosexual abuse of children of both genders occurs, as does involvement of children with combinations of adult partners. One young boy's promiscuous bisexual mother found it amusing to force his mouth upon the genitals of her lovers of both sexes. Another young girl's father regularly abused his six children, and had them perform mutual oral sex in a "daisy chain" fashion.

Physiological abuses occur when parents or caretakers engage in practices inconsistent with a child's age or actual needs. Probably the most common physiological abuses are those of "overcleaning," especially the "cleaning out" of infants through the use of laxatives and enemas. Not infrequently, a member of the family gives the infant or child adult doses of medication. As an example, an eight-month-old female infant received adult doses of barbiturates so she would sleep through the night and not bother the family. Most of her preschool years were spent in lethargy or actual sleep.

Psychological abuses are extraordinarily common. They consist of the inappropriate demeaning, denigrating, ridiculing, criticizing, and condemning of children, as well as placing them in intolerable situations that force them to accept double binds or gross distortions of reality (1, 2). Apart from the more gross and obvious abuses, there are many of a more subtle nature. When children ask for an adult's attention, particularly for some creative project or activity, the adult's failure to respond with interest and approval can be demoralizing. Frequently, adults make fun of or diminish a child's efforts, because they are at a childish level, without appreciating that they should be childish. Also, punishing infants or children for activities that are undesirable, but new, without explaining that the new activity is inappropriate and must not be repeated, is also unsettling, punitive, and frightening. Lasting injuries to self-worth and self-esteem result from these mistreatments.

Physicians and others commonly recognize physical abuse because bruises, broken bones, and other signs of tissue injury offer testimony of the harm that has been endured. In this context, I will only add that much physical abuse leaves no permanent trace, and many children receive no medical attention when wounds are fresh. Many children regularly miss school while bruises, burns, and black eyes heal at home; other children's wounds are misrepresented as the sequelae of accidents. Physiological abuse and psychological abuse invariably accompany physical abuse. In Chapter 3 of this monograph, Drs. Braun and Sachs will elaborate further on the types of abuse.

EFFECTS OF ABUSE ON THE PSYCHE

The effects on the psyche of the various kinds of child abuse are multitudinous. The outcome may depend upon the abused individual's genetic endowment and the response of persons in the individual's environment to the abuse; upon the types and sources of the abuse; upon the age of the individual and the number of years over which the abuse was endured; and upon the child's management of the tasks of various developmental stages. Because all of these factors must be taken into account, no single syndrome uniformly results from mistreatment. Child abuse has been correlated with psychoses, severe psychoneuroses, character disorders, borderline states, sociopathy, and possible criminality, as well as multiple personality disorder.

The examples of the types of abuses cited above were reported to my colleagues and me in the course of our work with multiple personality disorder patients. The majority of patients who develop multiple personality disorder have been victims of child abuse. Ninety-seven of 100 patients reviewed in a recent study had backgrounds of abuse (3). This underlines the importance of child abuse as an etiological factor, and the importance of its prevention.

Without abuse, we would have few cases of multiple personality disorder. A few children do dissociate due to terrifying accidents, serious illness, and a scattering of miscellaneous causes etiologically associated with this disorder (4). The eight-month-old girl who received adult doses of barbiturates throughout her infancy suffered many other abuses. In addition to her multiple personality disorder, this early physiological abuse left her with permanently disrupted sleep rhythms.

Another girl, a toddler, received adult doses of harsh cathartics, which resulted in several days of diarrhea. She had been expected to develop bowel continence quite prematurely, and when she could not control her bowels perfectly during the diarrheal episodes, she received severe corporal punishment.

Still another youngster who went on to develop multiple personality disorder was a nine-year-old boy who was buried in the ground by his stepfather. The stepfather put a stove pipe over his face so he could breathe. Of course, the boy became frantic. He screamed and cried. As he became still more upset, the stepfather threatened to leave him and to tell everyone he had run away. The boy's screams became louder. His stepfather told him to "Shut up." When the boy, out of control with terror, continued to scream, the stepfather voided into the stove pipe over the boy's face. The boy was not physically injured, but this demeaning and terrifying ordeal inflicted massive psychological abuse.

Development of Multiple Personality Disorder

Since multiple personality disorder is a mode of survival for some individuals who are capable of dissociating in the face of severe infant and child abuse, there is often a relationship between certain abuses and specific alternate personalities (5). Each alternate personality usually deals with a related set of conflicts and affects. Alternations or switches can occur when overwhelming feelings and conflicts are present as a result of the abuses. Subsequently, situations analogous to the abusive situations (which cause fear that abuse or some related harm might occur, or which stimulate an affect related to a particular alternate) may trigger switching.

For example, an alternate may deal only with hostile affects and conflicts that concern rage, anger, and hostility. This is quite a common finding in female multiple personality disorder patients who, as youngsters, were punished severely when they became angry, and were informed that their expression of anger proved that they were sinful, and would go to hell. In the several cases known to me, the young girls came to the conclusion that they must not express anger or rage. Consequently, these patients suppressed their feelings, although they knew these feelings were present. In making the effort to suppress the affect, they appeared to be "clouding up," or to be in a trance. They were then punished physically for looking distracted, and told that this behavior was not acceptable. They then completely repressed the hostile affects, no longer consciously coping with the pressure to control them (6).

Some examples will illustrate the outcomes. One patient, first seen as an adult, stated that she did not remember ever getting angry in her entire life. However, she had two alternates who dealt with rage, anger, hostility, and the anxiety associated with these feelings.

Another patient was overwhelmed by the amount, intensity, and duration of her rage reactions. They caused her severe anxiety.

She developed two alternates, one of whom dealt with the rage, and another who dealt with the anxiety about the rage.

A third patient developed a violent personality when, at the age of 4½, she discovered that she could make her abusive stepfather, who was coming after her, back away when she had a large carving knife in her hand. The hostile alternate carried a weapon with her from then on, always on guard against an overwhelming attack by her stepfather, whom she feared would kill her by "stomping" her.

Another patient developed an alternate violent personality that embodied the rage he felt when his stepfather abused him sexually. This alternate later was arrested for severely beating a homosexual who had made advances toward him.

Still another patient, known in the literature as "Jonah" (7), developed a violent personality when he was set upon by three boys larger than himself. He thought they were going to kill him. The personality that had sustained the initial onslaught retreated. The violent personality that emerged was so frightening and fought with such ferocity that the three larger boys ran away. Thereafter, this hostile alternate believed he could not be injured or bested in any situation. He appeared so omnipotent that when he was interviewed in a hospital setting, many psychiatrists interpreted the omnipotence as the delusional grandiosity of schizophrenia. A careful review of the origins of this personality, however, shows that he had some "basis" for feeling omnipotent. Not only had he driven away three larger boys when he was seven years of age, but also, while in control of the body during combat in Viet Nam, he had survived the numerous dangerous missions for which he volunteered; and, in addition, he recovered from a wound. He finally was removed from combat and sent stateside after this personality, while manning a machine gun, succeeded not only in pinning down the enemy, but in pinning down his own forces as well. The original or birth personality had no recollection of ever having been in combat. In fact, he did not remember ever having been outside of the United States. In contrast, the hostile alternate could detail his experience in the war zone without difficulty.

Alternates may also be formed to deal with sexual affects and the conflicts resulting from sexual abuses (7). One woman had been raped by her father when she was 4½ years of age, and subsequently was used as a sexual object not only by her father, but also by some of his friends. At the time of the rape she developed a very passive alternate who allowed this type of abuse to continue. She had learned that if she dared to resist, she suffered severe physical abuse, as well as sexual violation. Ironically, the father and his friends considered the girl's passivity as a sign that she enjoyed their sexual use of her—after all, she never resisted. They indulged themselves without hesitation or guilt.

Another female patient had a father who attempted to seduce her with sex play and then raped her shortly before her fourth birthday. At this time, she developed two hostile alternates. One was a boy whose only set of feelings dealt with his interest in killing the little girl's father. The second was also a hostile alternate, but it kept the homicidal little boy under control, and preserved the sexual affects.

Alternates may come into existence to preserve a biological function or to preserve a talent that is felt to be threatened by the abuser. One little girl was very musical and loved to play the piano. She refused to play any more after her mother threatened to break her fingers if she made any more mistakes. She never played in the presence of another person again; but an alternate, created to preserve the love of music, would hurry to the piano and play for hours when the girl was entirely alone in the house. No other human being ever heard her play.

One young man, who was arrested for rape, was discovered to have a large number of alternate personalities, one of whom was a late adolescent female whose sexual orientation was lesbian. Investigation discovered that this alternate had been in control of the body at the time of the rape. The birth personality had retreated two years before the rape. When that personality had been active, he had dated a young lady steadily. However, he was totally impotent when he and his girlfriend attempted sexual relations. It emerged that all the male personalities in the man's complex of alternates had experienced their own sexual abuse during childhood as so devastating, terrifying, and painful that they experienced themselves as incapable of normal sexual function. The lesbian female alternate preserved sexuality. She felt that she had never been abused. Tragically, her preservation of sexuality achieved expression in what took the form of a sexual assault.

A male alternate in a female patient appeared to deal with her overwhelming fear of her grandfather. This man was a large blustering individual who was abusive of his small-statured wife, the patient's grandmother. The child and her parents lived in the same building, but not in the same apartment. She adored her grandmother and disliked her grandfather for his mistreatment of her. She was forced to spend a lot of time around her grandfather, who not only menaced her grandmother, but vociferously and arrogantly berated everyone he encountered or spoke about: everyone was "evil" and sure to wind up in hell. The grandfather built a doll house for the little girl and had her help him. She was so terrified of him she could neither work with him nor enjoy the doll house, except through a male alternate, who identified with grandfather. Note that this is an example of the formation of an alternate by identification with an aggressor.

It is possible to offer a theoretical construct to explain the alternation of personalities and the occurrence of multiple personality disorder. Abuses create in the child a state of an unacceptable and threatening feeling: for example, rage. The child learns that the feeling is unacceptable, and that it must not only be unexpressed, but it must not even be consciously "felt." The feeling or affect is repressed and remains in the unconscious, outside of awareness (9). Individuals who repress affects in this manner seem to build up a "bank" of feeling that creates a potential for explosions of that feeling when repression breaks down. These explosions of feeling may be expressed in some symptomatic fashion. When the repression of feeling is accompanied by conflicts (both in relation to that particular feeling, and with regard to related other feelings that are also repressed), the combined presence of the overwhelming affects and the serious conflicts (both of which have been repressed) may result in the emergence of an alternate personality as a vehicle for the symptomatic expression of these affects and associated conflicts.

Physical Symptoms Associated With Multiple Personality Disorder

Multiple personality disorder is defined by the presence of alternate personalities; but as a clinical entity, it is often characterized by a multitude of psychosomatic disturbances and hysterical symptoms as well. When one alternate manifests a functional symptom or suffers a psychosomatic condition and other alternates do not, the discrepancy may serve as a valuable clue toward discovering the emotional conflicts involved in the dynamics of that particular alternate. Similarly, when a conversion symptom or psychosomatic flare-up occurs in a particular alternate whose unique conflicts, affects, and concerns are already known, the interplay between the symptomatic events, the dynamics, and the traumata underlying them may be clarified rapidly.

An example of a physical symptom associated with repressed rage was a woman's recurrent diarrhea following a situation in which she was entitled to become enraged, yet had no awareness of that affect.

Migraine headaches are experienced by many patients suffering multiple personality disorder. Some are precipitated by repressed rage. Others occur when one alternate punishes or intrudes upon another, or when one tries to escape from an undesirable situation that is buried in the unconscious. One patient noted the onset of a migraine episode. Upon questioning, an alternate said she was going to have to face an undesirable social situation. Exploration revealed that the birth personality did not know she could refuse to be involved: that she could and should say "no." When both personalities became convinced it was possible to say "no," the incipient migraine was cut short.

Effects of Multiple Personality Disorder on Society

Many persons who suffer multiple personality disorder are

bright and talented. Their abuse as infants and children can produce horrifying results. Decompensated multiple personality disorder patients may lose access to their skills or training, become unable to use talents and intelligence, and experience frightening episodes of time loss; that is, amnesia. The patients' loss of health, opportunities, and access to their natural ability to learn and profit from education, seriously compromise their abilities to live, love, and work.

Not only does society lose the constructive contributions of bright, talented individuals; in some cases, multiple personality disorder patients develop alternates that channel their intelligence and creativity into the expression of hostility and aggression, and become involved in major and occasionally violent crimes. The violent criminal outcome (an infrequent and far from typical consequence) offers a poignant illustration of the profound social cost of child abuse, and the severe and protracted mental illnesses that it can create. The overall expense to society of the crimes committed by this minority of the total multiple personality disorder patient group is imposing: they are lost as productive citizens; their victims suffer; and the price of arrest, trial, and incarceration must be born. Once arrested and confined, it is unlikely that these individuals will either be diagnosed or receive the intensive therapy that could bring about the change that might remove them from the pool of recidivist criminals.

TREATMENT OF MULTIPLE PERSONALITY DISORDER

Psychiatrists and nonphysician therapists who have worked extensively with multiple personality disorder patients express optimism about their prospects for recovery (4). However, they state that recovery is contingent upon the availability of specially trained clinicians who understand the condition thoroughly. In the course of treatment, it is necessary for the therapist to explain the condition to the patient, so that the patient can understand his or her circumstances and begin to deal therapeutically with the alternation of personalities. In my experience, multiple personality disorder patients' cooperation is excellent when they comprehend what has been happening in their lives. Very few who find themselves in an adequate treatment with a competent, knowledgeable therapist drop out of therapy. Almost all go on to fusion and recovery. My experience is confirmed by Kluft's follow-up studies (4).

In the course of treating such patients, one frequently hears distressing stories of their futile attempts to seek help as children. In one case, noted earlier, a child who was sexually abused by her father and his friends went to a counselor for help when she was 11 years of age. The counselor believed the child, and was extremely upset by the detailed report that the child had given her. She told the child that she would investigate the situation and would do what she could to help her. This young counselor, a social worker, was apparently unable to obtain any confirming information. Her supervisor told her repeatedly that the child was probably dealing with her own fantasies in relation to her father and his friends. The counselor found herself unable to give the child any concrete assistance, although she talked to the child on many occasions over a two-year period, and remained convinced that the child was being truthful.

Another patient had a father who beat her regularly and condemned her to hell. This man was a minister, whose hypocrisy allowed him to rationalize his extreme abusiveness. There were many public evidences of his mistreatment of both the patient and his wife, but no one in the church or community was prepared to believe that the minister could possibly be abusive.

CONCLUSION

Several multiple personality disorder patients have complained bitterly that child abuse starts with society's approval of the spanking of children. They report that they were frequently spanked so hard, they were left covered with bruises. As we have seen in some of the case examples cited in this chapter, they report that their parents offered bizarre rationalizations for their excessive corporal punishment (such as the patient whose mother told her, "I can hit you as hard as I wish on your bottom because it has no feelings").

Unfortunately, the sanctioning of physical punishment, even if severe, is only one of several factors that lead to the minimizing of accusations of child abuse. School counselors and social workers often receive reports of child abuse that they believe are due to fantasy, and decide against investigating. Also, abused children often are fearful of reporting their mistreatment, especially if the abuse began early in life. Furthermore, small children may report that they were hurt by "monsters," which actually represent an abusive parent or relative.

When abuse charges enter the legal system, it is rare that abusive parents give accurate accounts of their actions. Usually, they deny any misdeeds, understate the severity of the punishments they have imposed, and offer plausible explanations that represent the child as a liar who requires "discipline." Some judges may ask the parents to seek treatment of some sort, and send the child back to the abusive home. In fact, many abusive parents promptly drop out of treatment. The legal system's follow-up is often nonexistent. The abusive family, however, is likely to inflict still further severe abuse in retaliation for its brush with the legal system.

Belief systems that encourage the use of physical punishment in order to discipline a child and bring him or her up to be a responsible adult often imply permission, under the banner of "Spare the rod, spoil the child," to employ excessive corporal force. The children often identify with this value system. In many abusive families there is an additional conspiracy of silence. The children are brought up hearing the order "Don't tell!" Thus, adequate information is difficult to acquire; information that is obtained may be understated and revealed with great guilt.

This chapter has focused on multiple personality disorder and its relationship to child abuse. However, many instances of psychoses, borderline states, psychoneuroses, sociopathy, and criminal behaviors in general are also associated with the mistreatment of children. It would behoove us as a society to reverse our unfortunate tendency to disregard accounts of abuses suffered by infants, children, and adolescents. To appreciate, understand, and listen to the communications of young people is a vitally important first step in the prevention of these disturbances in our future adult population.

References

1. Summit RC: The child abuse accommodation syndrome. Child Abuse Negl 7:177-193, 1983

2. Kluft RP, Braun BG, Sachs R: Multiple personality, intrafamilial abuse, and family psychiatry. International Journal of Family Psychiatry (in press)

3. Putnam FW, Post RM, Guroff JJ, et al: One hundred cases of multiple personality disorder. Presented at the Annual Meeting of the American Psychiatric Association, New Research Abstract #77, New York, 1983

4. Kluft RP: Treatment of multiple personality disorder. Psychiatr Clin North Am 7:9-29, 1984

5. Kluft RP: The epidemiology of multiple personality. Paper presented at Multiple Personality: Finding and Fusing, a course at the Annual Meeting of the American Psychiatric Association, Chicago, May, 1979

6. Ellenberger HF: The Discovery of the Unconscious. New York, Basic Books, 1980

7. Ludwig AM, Brandsma JM, Wilbur CB, et al: The objective study of a multiple personality, or, are four heads better than one? Arch Gen Psychiatry 26:298-310, 1972

8. Allison RB: A guide to parents: how to raise your daughter to have multiple personalities. Family Therapy 1:83-88, 1974

9. Wilbur CB: Treatment of multiple personality. Psychiatric Annals 14:27-31, 1984

3

The Development of Multiple Personality Disorder: Predisposing, Precipitating, and Perpetuating Factors

Bennett G. Braun, M.D., M.S.
Roberta G. Sachs, Ph.D.

3

The Development of Multiple Personality Disorder: Predisposing, Precipitating, and Perpetuating Factors

Multiple personality disorder has received increasing attention in the last three decades. This renewed interest has been spurred by books such as *The Three Faces of Eve* (1) and *Sybil* (2), and their adaptation into well-received movies. The current Diagnostic and Statistical Manual of Mental Disorders, Third Edition (DSM-III) recognizes multiple personality disorder as a syndrome distinct from the hysterical disorders (3).

Many new studies have expanded our understanding of this disorder substantially; new forums have become available for the sharing of knowledge and exploration of the topic's frontiers. Four journals have dedicated recent issues to the study of multiple personality disorder (*American Journal of Clinical Hypnosis*, Volume 26:2, 1983; *Psychiatric Annals*, Volume 14:1, 1984; *Psychiatric Clinics of North America*, Volume 7:1, 1984; *International Journal of Clinical and Experimental Hypnosis*, Volume 32:2, 1984). The First International Conference on Multiple Personality/Dissociative States was held in Chicago in September, 1984. This chapter will attempt to systematize and integrate current clinical observations and research data in order to summarize and conceptualize ideas being studied in the growing literature on multiple personality disorder.

A useful heuristic model for the study of any psychiatric

disorder involves the consideration of the predisposing, precipitating, and perpetuating factors that accompany its symptomatic manifestations. By studying the predisposing factors, we can, it is hoped, identify those stimuli that render the individual susceptible to developing a particular disorder. These factors include both genetic and environmental variables. By examining the precipitating event(s), we attempt to understand those variables that trigger the onset of the clinical disorder. Finally, by studying the perpetuating phenomena, we can observe the contingencies that maintain the behavioral, psychological, and physiological manifestations of the disorder.

We will begin with a brief description of multiple personality disorder. This will be followed by three sections. These will focus, respectively, on the predisposing, precipitating, or perpetuating factors that correspond to the development of this disorder. Next, we will present two brief case histories in order to illustrate how the preceding sections contribute to a greater understanding of the course of this syndrome. We will conclude with a brief summary and some suggestions for future research.

THE PHENOMENON OF MULTIPLE PERSONALITY DISORDER

The phenomenon of multiple personality disorder was first reported almost four centuries ago (4). Ellenberger (5) offers a superb summary of cases reported from before 1800, through to the 1950s. Cases reported by Janet (6) and Prince (7) attracted wide attention to this syndrome at the end of the 19th and the beginning of the 20th century. It is impossible to estimate the incidence of multiple personality disorder in the days of Janet and Prince. Relevant data was not collected, and accurate records are not available. Even if we had such reports, we could not be sure whether some of these cases would be better understood as other entities, in light of current knowledge and diagnostic classifications.

However, it seems clear that after a flurry of interest in this condition, there was a dramatic decline in the number of cases reported in the years immediately following Bleuler's introduction of the diagnostic entity of "schizophrenia" (around 1910). Some have suggested that many multiple personality disorder patients have been misdiagnosed as schizophrenics since this date (8). Others have proposed that the post-1910 decline of interest in this syndrome was spurred by the view that the symptoms of multiple personality disorder were an artifact of hypnotic suggestion (9). It was not until the dramatic cases of "Eve" (1) and "Sybil" (2) had aroused the attention of the professional community (as well as lay audiences) that investigators began to consider that multiple personality disorder was distinguishable from schizophrenia (8) and was not an artifact of hypnotic suggestion (10, 11). Current attempts to estimate the incidence and prevalence of multiple personality disorder are still plagued by a lack of consensus regarding the etiology and the descriptive boundaries of the syndrome.

Multiple personality disorder is one of five dissociative disorders delineated in the current DSM-III. The common feature of all dissociative disorders is a spontaneous and temporary fluctuation in the normal integrative functions and consciousness. In multiple personality disorder, this feature manifests itself as a temporary alteration in awareness of one's identity. Instead of sustaining an ongoing continuity of identity, afflicted individuals may assume a new identity or personality. Often, an alter personality will be aware of the original or "host" personality. However, the "host" personality usually claims to be unaware of the existence of other personalities. In addition, information acquired while the other personalities had executive control of the body may not be accessible to the "host" personality. The contemporary picture of multiple personality disorder was recently summarized by Kluft, who compiled a glossary of terms used by contemporary workers (12).

There are three diagnostic criteria for multiple personality disorder in DSM-III: 1) the existence within an individual of two (or more) distinct personalities, each of which is in control of the body at different times; 2) the personality that is dominant determines ongoing behavior; and 3) each personality is complex and has its own unique history, behavior patterns, and social relationships. While these criteria form a beginning foundation for the reliable identification of multiple personality disorder, they do not address the issues regarding the construct of "dissociation," which most workers consider essential to a thorough appreciation of the etiology, dynamics, and treatment of the condition. Dissociation is far too broad and complex a subject for extensive treatment here. A brief and, necessarily, selective commentary is offered.

Janet is usually credited with developing the "classical" concept of "dissociation"; it seems reasonable to infer that this exegesis was influenced by his clinical observation of multiple personality disorder patients. He believed that consciousness was not a unitary phenomenon. Rather, he thought, it flowed in streams that did not necessarily intersect. Hence, information entering consciousness via one stream did not always flow or find its way into another stream. This metaphor seemed to offer an adequate explanation for many of the symptomatic manifestations of multiple personality disorder.

Recent theorizing about dissociation (13) has proposed some modifications of Janet's concepts. For example, some investigators have drawn parallels between dissociation and hypnosis (13–15); state-dependent learning (16), and current neuropsychophysiological models of synaptic transmission (17). These new formulations have offered increased specificity regarding the processes involved in dissociation without detracting from the broad explanatory power of Janet's original model.

Recent studies using standardized hypnotizability scales have demonstrated that multiple personality disorder patients are more hypnotizable than are other clinical populations (14, 18). This finding has been replicated and expanded by investigators who used examiners blind to the patients' diagnoses at the time of testing (19). A number of workers had anticipated these findings, either on theoretical grounds or by relying on impressionistic clinical estimations of hypnotizability (11, 15, 20–22). Related studies, based on the analysis of case reports, clearly indicate that information acquired while one personality is in executive control of the body is still available to the system, although it may not be consciously accessible to other personalities at a given point in time (13, 20). Silberman has demonstrated this phenomenon in a controlled research setting (23).

In summary, much additional research is needed to clarify the explanatory powers of several alternative, but largely overlapping, models of "dissociation." It is hoped that investigations will focus on dissociation in both clinical and experimental contexts in order to resolve remaining questions. For the present, however, until controlled laboratory research becomes feasible and its results both replicable and rendered accessible, we are constrained to interpret and extrapolate from clinical observations. These clinical observations appear to establish the course of multiple personality disorder as unique from other syndromes.

PREDISPOSING FACTORS

Clinical observations made systematically over the last few years have identified two major predisposing factors for multiple personality disorder. These factors are: 1) a natural, inborn capacity to dissociate; and 2) exposure to severe, overwhelming traumata, such as frequent, unpredictable, and inconsistently alternating abuse and love (especially during childhood). Both of these factors, taken together, are hypothesized to be a necessary cause of multiple personality disorder; but neither factor alone is sufficient to cause this disorder. We will examine each factor separately.

Inborn Capacity to Dissociate

Many current investigators have hypothesized that the mal-adaptive ability to dissociate is an integral or main cause of multiple personality disorder (4, 11, 15, 17). However, this hypothesis is not new. It can be traced to Janet's seminal contributions (6). Prince also discussed this possible explanation (7). The main difference between earlier conceptions and current formulations is that in the latter, it is recognized that dissociation of consciousness occurs only or predominantly at the level of awareness. That is, in many cases, information acquired when another personality has executive control over the body can still affect behavior when the host personality has control (13). The information acquired by the alternate personality (or personalities) can exert an unconscious or semiconscious influence on the host personality's ongoing behavior; while the host, consciously in control, remains unaware of the influence being exerted upon it.

The ability to dissociate has been proposed to have biological determinants (10, 15, 17). Although no twin studies have yet been undertaken to test this hypothesis, evidence now exists that the incidence of multiple personality disorder may be transgenerational (see Chapter 6 of this monograph). While these preliminary observations are more suggestive than conclusive and are subject to numerous criticisms (some might feel they "beg the question"; others might see them as tautological), they lend some support to the hypothesis that there may be a genetic factor to dissociation. There is also some evidence that responsivity to hypnosis may also be genetically determined (24). Frischholz (in Chapter 5 of this monograph) critically evaluates this evidence and its potential heuristic value for understanding multiple personality disorder.

The relation between hypnosis and dissociation has been alluded to briefly in an earlier section. Over five decades of empirical research has clearly demonstrated that a classical dissociation explanation of hypnotic phenomena falls short of offering a comprehensive explication (24–29). In most of the relevant experiments, the subjects learn something and are then instructed to have post-hypnotic amnesia for what was learned. In brief, these experiments show that when subjects are tested on the material that has been learned and hypnotically dissociated, this dissociated material appears to exert an influence on the test performance of these subjects that is not found in otherwise comparable subjects who have never before been exposed to the material in any manner.

Hilgard has offered a recent revision of the classical concept of dissociation (13). In his reformulation, the keeping of dissociated information from awareness requires some type of separate cognitive structure and activity. While the information may exert some influence on overt behavior, it should only be considered dissociated if the subject reports being unaware of both it and its effect. This reformulation per se, called "neodissociation theory," is consistent with the type of dissociation observed in clinical work with multiple personality disorder patients. For example, multiple personality disorder patients are more likely to experience the hidden observer phenomenon described by Hilgard (13), and the phenomenon of dualism in age regressions, than are other patient groups. Both of these hypnotic phenomena are assumed to be forms of dissociation. They appear to offer new perspectives for examining the relationship between hypnosis and dissociation. However, it must be acknowledged that evidence for the universal presence of the cognitive structures and activities that Hilgard described is neither invariably obvious nor straightforward in all cases of multiple personality disorder.

Memory, Intelligence, and Creativity

Most individuals with multiple personality disorder have several additional features that operate in relation to the ability to dissociate: an excellent working memory, above-average intelligence, and creativity. A good "working memory" is necessary in multiple personality disorder, because the knowledge that is accumulated by the various personalities must be kept separated in the memory. Yet this separation is by no means complete in all respects, nor is the type of separation uniform. Ellenberger has described many patterns (5). Some personalities have access to some of the data collected by the other personalities (one-way amnesia) (30). The various structures of this selective interpersonality sharing of information must be remembered in order to be maintained.

Characteristically, most multiple personality disorder patients show evidence of having above-average intelligence, although this may not be accompanied by outstanding performances on standard intelligence tests. In the present discussion, we speak of intelligence as an adaptive ability, following Garcia's descriptions and discussions (31). The symptoms of multiple personality disorder argue against using a score on a particular IQ test as an operational definition of intelligence with this patient group. It is not uncommon to learn, retrospectively, that a child personality may have had control of the body during one particular testing session. Thus, the test results for a grown adult may give the appearance of unrealistically poor functioning, even mental retardation. During another session for the same patient, an adult personality may have control of the body and the person's performance on an IQ test could jump as much as 40 to 50 points.

There does not seem to be an acceptable method for determining the overall IQ of a multiple personality disorder patient with a single test. A more revealing use of IQ tests in understanding multiple personality disorder would be to do repeated IQ testings of several adult and child personalities. Analysis of both the inter- and intrapersonality IQ test correlations would provide data about whether these personalities were structurally consistent with regard to IQ.

Defining intelligence as the ability to adapt to one's environment is consistent with both Binet's and Wechsler's conceptualization of this construct (32). The adaptive function of the symptomatology of multiple personality disorder becomes more obvious when one considers that multiple personality disorder patients are exposed to events that produce anxiety overwhelming enough to cause a psychotic decompensation in most normal people. The dissociative defense becomes maladaptive when there is a lack of discrimination between a stressful and a traumatic event, and disproportionate responses are mobilized. For example, in one instance a patient, as a child, developed an alternate aggressive personality in order to defend itself against an abusing parent. This use of the dissociative defense proved adaptive, and was reinforced by success in terminating the abuse. However, when the patient, in adult life, could not discriminate between abuse and minor criticism from other authority figures, and an aggressive personality emerged in order to protect itself against what it misperceived as a potentially overwhelming threat, the dissociative response became maladaptive.

The last characteristic related to an inborn capacity to dissociate is creativity. This should not seem very surprising, since the psychological system in multiple personality disorder patients in a sense "created" the alternate personalities. However, this creativity often emerges through artistic or poetic expression. For example, art critics have noted that the paintings and drawings done by "Sybil" were good enough to display in prestigious art galleries. The authors have also seen multiple personality disorder cases where the patients were accomplished sculptors, poets, and composers.

Child Abuse

In addition to the ability to dissociate, and the features of memory, intelligence and creativity, another major predisposing factor for multiple personality disorder is inconsistent and unpredictable exposure to some form of traumatic abuse (33). Usually, this maltreatment begins in early childhood and extends through adolescence. The abuse can take many forms (such as neglect, physical punishment, psychological debasement, sexual abuse, and so forth), is usually unprovoked, and often takes many bizarre forms (34).

Sachs et al. (33) explain some of the differences between child abuse victims who have and have not developed multiple personality disorder. For example, nonmultiple personality disorder child abuse victims with a relative lack of dissociative ability usually have some type of sexual dysfuncton (such as frigidity or impotence). However, multiple personality disorder patients who were victims of child abuse always have some form of sexuality present in their system of personalities. Another difference between these two groups concerns the ability to experience joy or pleasure. Nonmultiple personality disorder child abuse victims are frequently anhedonic. In contrast, child abuse victims who developed multiple personality disorder are still able to experience happiness and pleasure in their ongoing lives. These capacities are preserved by some personalities.

Sachs et al. (33) propose that the reason some child abuse victims develop multiple personality disorder while others do not is moderated by individual differences in the capacity to dissociate. Nonmultiple personality disorder child abuse victims who lack this dissociative ability defend against this abuse by supression and denial. However, child abuse victims who do possess a strong dissociative potential utilize this ability in the face of continuing stress. Thus, the major difference between child abuse victims who do and do not develop multiple personality disorder is based on the degree to which the ability to dissociate is available in their biological repertoire of responses.

In order to promote the development of multiple personality disorder, the abuse must be frequent, unpredictable, and inconsistent. The child is also exposed to some form of love. Infrequent maltreatment will lead to sporadic dissociative episodes that do not take on a life history of their own. Only when such abuse is frequent and inconsistently repetitive do the dissociative episodes begin to coalesce into a personality. Chronic abuse stimulates repeated dissociations which, when chained together by a shared affective state, develop into a personality with a unique identity and behavioral repertoire (10, 17).

The nature of the maltreatment to which the child is exposed also distinguishes the general abuse victim from the child who will develop multiple personality disorder. This distinction is not absolute, however. Child abuse victims who do not develop multiple personality disorder are more frequently subject to reactive aggression on the part of their parents. Multiple personality disorder child abuse victims, on the other hand, are usually subject to sadistic and bizarre abuse in addition to, or without, reactive aggression. This mistreatment often is ritualistic and driven by the abuser's own motivations. One male multiple personality disorder patient was subjected to the following ritual: the patient's mother used to insert pearls into the penile urethra. She pushed a pearl on a thread into the urethra with a thermometer and then pulled it out. The occurrence of the abuses to which this and other multiple personality disorder patients were exposed was often inconsistent with the parental behaviors that had immediately preceded the parent's aggression. For example, a child may be told by his mother, "I love you," and then burned with a cigarette.

Child abuse has been found to be a transgenerational problem (35). This haunting observation may be related to the transgenerational nature of multiple personality disorder, discussed by Braun in Chapter 6 of this monograph. Certainly, the incidence of child abuse seems to be very much greater in the families of multiple personality disorder patients than in normals (33). Future research should address whether the occurrence of child abuse in the histories of multiple personality disorder patients is significantly greater than is the incidence of child abuse in other clinical groups.

PRECIPITATING FACTORS

A precipitating factor is one that can be identified as being antecedent to the initiation of a set of intrapsychic processes and structures that lead to the formation of a new personality. The diagnosis of multiple personality disorder is usually made long after the personalities become separate (12). It may be difficult at that time to determine what were the specific precipitating factors in many of the divisions. Furthermore, a patient in therapy may form new, short-lived entities in response to aspects of treatment, especially in order to deny recovered memories and to encapsulate hospitalizations.

This may appear to leave the issue of personality formation confused. The dissociation process is facilitated with experience, and fragments may later be created with relative ease over relatively less stressful episodes. However, it is essential to refrain from reasoning retrospectively that because later personality or fragment formations may be triggered by relatively minor stressors, the stressors that initiated the disorder were trivial. Recently, Kluft reported on a youngster assessed before and after abuse. He noted the youngster's development of multiple personality disorder shortly after the abuse began (see Chapter 8 of this monograph). This and anterospective studies under way (see Chapter 4 of this monograph) give credence to long-held clinical impressions, derived from patients' retrospective accounts.

Undoubtedly, the most common of the factors linked to the precipitation of multiple personality disorder is some form of abuse that triggers defensive dissociative episodes. Other etiologies have been reported (Chapters 4 and 6 of this monograph; 14, 17, 20, 36, 38). Any type of abuse (for example, physical, emotional, or sexual) may bring this about, as long as it is sufficiently traumatic. Dissociation then may become the chief defense to provide some relief from the horror of the abuse. This is especially true when the predisposing factors are in place.

It is also difficult to identify the initial dissociative episode, since there is no objective method for checking the validity of the information. However, there is now enough evidence to show that some individuals begin defensively dissociating from distress felt at two or three years of age (37–40). Some patients report beginning at even younger ages. The exact specification of which abusive incident occurred first is perhaps less important than how the series of dissociated states gradually gains structure.

The formation of an alternate personality occurs when a series of fragmented but defensively related episodes, linked by a common affective state, take on an identity of their own. This usually happens when the series of episodes are conceptually related to a particular type of event. At this point, an analogy between computers and multiple personality disorder becomes useful (17). It is almost as if two separate memory systems are created. Memory System "A" contains information that forms the identity of the "host" personality. Memory System "B," which is split off from Memory System "A," contains that information which system A was unwilling or unable to integrate. This information can be centered around a common theme, such as anger toward authority (parental) figures, developmentally conflictual drives, or opposing emotions. The structurally organizing theme of these previously fragmented episodes now gives the new entity an identity and purpose. In the case of anger toward authority figures, this new personality may pop up whenever the host personality feels he or she is pushed around by someone who is perceived as having some control over his or her life (for example, a boss, a wife, a best friend).

It is not unusual for Personality "A" to be further split into additional memory systems. This occurs whenever a series of related dissociative episodes become structurally organized into a coherent system, with a slightly different common theme or a different reaction to a common theme. Hence, other alternate personalities are born, each with their own defensive function (17). Sachs et al. (33) have commented on the parallels between the various personalities that exist in the multiple personality disorder patient and his or her family dynamics.

To summarize, in terms of understanding the development and organization of the separate personalities, it is most relevant to identify when a series of dissociative episodes become structurally organized by a unifying defensive theme into an alternate personality. The specific incidents that trigger the initial dissociations, and, as an aggregate, lead to personality formation, are often more crucial as events to be dealt with in therapy than as explanations of personality formation per se. A similar approach should be taken in understanding the genesis of other personalities. Each will have a particular purpose and will have memories associated with it. In some multiple personality disorder patients, the management of defensive themes has become so specialized that many personalities appear. The personalities that appear, and that have a range of emotions, memories, and behaviors, make up a system we call multiple personality disorder.

PERPETUATING FACTORS

The perpetuating factors in the course of multiple personality disorder have three main components: personal, interpersonal, and situational. The personal component concerns the observation that multiple personality disorder patients repeatedly use dissociation as a defense against stress. Since the dissociation usually results in a temporary relief from stress and anxiety, the repeated use of this ability as a coping mechanism leads to its being continuously reinforced. Hence, it becomes the preferred or dominant form of defense in the individual's psychological system.

The observation and treatment of childhood multiple personality disorder is one way to study the potential reinforcing value of using a dissociative defense. For example, we would expect that the personalities that appear in childhood multiple personality disorder would be less developed than personalities observed in an adult multiple personality disorder patient. Similarly, we would expect that it would be easier to teach childhood multiple personality disorder patients alternate coping strategies than it would be to teach adult multiple personality disorder patients these strategies, because the reinforcing value of the dissociative defensive style has had a shorter life history in children. This is consistent with Kluft's findings in actual cases of childhood multiple personality disorder (36, 39).

The interpersonal factors that continue to perpetuate the symptomatic manifestations of multiple personality disorder are varied, but usually relate to the patient's family dynamics. It is understandable that the cause of dissociative splitting should also contribute to its perpetuation. As an example, we will continue to elaborate on the theme of anger toward authority figures. This construct is usually the organizing theme of a series of dissociative episodes. These episodes were related, because they all involved early abusive incidents in which an authority figure (usually a parent) took part. Since the host could not express the rage that it felt when abused by the authority figure, the rage was split off and the task of its acknowledgement or expression was left to the alternate personality that had developed in response to this need. However, stimulus generalization occurs, and all authority figures become perceived as abusive. Therefore, whenever the host personality is unable to express its anger, the alternate personality takes over and may express this affect in an extreme or inappropriate manner. Since this defense has yielded temporary relief in the past, it is used frequently. This can be very maladaptive when the authority figure who triggers the switching is the patient's spouse or boss.

Situational variables that perpetuate the development of multiple personality disorder include direct exposure to traumatic events, as well as the more indirect effect of societal attitudes and pressures. For example, in one multiple personality disorder case, the deaths of several family members within a short period promoted the development of alternate personalities in order to cope with serially overwhelming anxieties that centered around a common theme. In another case, the patient was continuously forced to accompany her homicidal brother, and actually witnessed several bizarre ritualistic murders. This patient reported many details about these crimes during treatment both to her therapist and then to the police. These details were later verified; they had never before been reported publicly, and the patient had no other obvious connection to the killings. These considerations corroborated the accuracy of the patient's account, and highlighted the way situational traumata had perpetuated the dissociative symptoms of multiple personality disorder.

Indirect situational perpetuating variables on the development of multiple personality disorder are more general societal influences, such as attitudes toward child care and discipline. For example, in some groups, the axiom "Spare the rod and spoil the child" is taken quite literally. In such circumstances, the parents may not understand their disciplinary actions as being abusive because other parents behave in the same way, and they believe they are helping their children. Despite such consensual validation and good intentions, the impact on a child so reared can be devastating.

Examples of the personal, interpersonal, and situational factors that perpetuate the symptomatic manifestations of multiple personality disorder will be discussed in the next section. These factors must be addressed in the treatment of any multiple personality disorder patient. The journey toward integration cannot begin until they are understood and mitigated.

DEVELOPMENT OF A MODEL FOR UNDERSTANDING MULTIPLE PERSONALITY DISORDER

Figure 1 summarizes the preceding discussion on the predisposing, precipitating, and perpetuating factors in the development of multiple personality disorder. The diagram presents a model that integrates previous theorizing about multiple personality disorder (10, 12, 36), child abuse (41), and dissociation (10, 17). An earlier version of this model has been presented elsewhere (34).

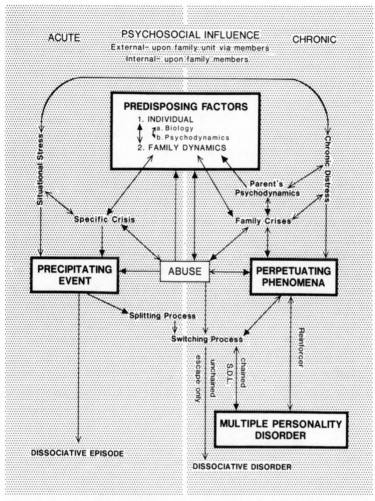

Figure 1. The influence of the three Ps (predisposing factors, precipitating events, and perpetuating phenomena) on the creation of multiple personality disorder. Solid arrowheads indicate a greater degree of influence than do open arrowheads.

At the top of the model are the psychosocial influences (direct and indirect) that go across the midline because they have both acute and chronic interactive effects on all of the other variables listed below (42). The predisposing factors include both individual (biological capacity to dissociate, individual psychodynamics) and environmental (family dynamics) variables. These factors interact with inconsistent love/abuse or other traumatic stimuli until one particular precipitating event causes an initial split. This is reinforcing because it protects the system from the overwhelming anxiety associated with the event. If sufficient perpetuating phenomena are present to stimulate repeated dissociation, an alternate personality begins to develop. Eventually, this cycle can lead to more dissociation and splitting, which may yield additional personalities, each of which has a particular adaptive function.

The flexibility of the model is evident in several ways. First, while abuse is a sufficient condition for triggering a dissociative split, it is not always necessary. The authors have reported an incidence of some type of child abuse in approximately 90 percent of the multiple personality disorder cases they have seen (33). This clearly indicates that abuse is not a factor in all multiple personality disorder cases. However, when abuse is absent, there is usually a history of some traumatic event that precipitated the initial dissociative split. Such events have included the death of a parent, a near-drowning, and frequent moves at an early age. The common link between inconsistent abuse and these traumatic stimuli is that both are events that are associated with overwhelming anxiety. These events, when accompanied by various perpetuating phenomena, are what initiate and promote the development of multiple personality disorder.

The arrows in Figure 1 that connect the different boxes signify a one-way cause, or a reciprocally determined influence. Bold arrow heads represent major effects in the model, while small arrowheads indicate lesser effects.

The heuristic value of the diagram lies in the fact that it can be used as a general nonmathematical model for understanding the development of multiple personality disorder while, at the same time, allowing the possibility of an ideographic analysis of a particular case. This will be illustrated in the next section. Two case examples will be presented, which highlight the value of this proposal. Each case will be discussed in reference to the model pictured in Figure 1.

Case Example 1

The first case is a 48-year-old female who was referred for treatment by another psychiatrist. He suspected she suffered multiple personality disorder. The diagnosis was confirmed (by B.G.B.), and treatment has continued over the last four years. The individual predisposing factors included her ability to dissociate. She was tested for hypnotizability on two well-accepted measures. Her score on a Stanford Form C (43) was 9/12. She received a 10/12 HIP Induction Score (15). Her ego structure included certain primitive defensive constellations.

This dissociative capacity is also evident in an older sister, whom she later referred for treatment of a depression. It is interesting to note that while the patient and her older sister were both exposed to the same set of circumstances and had similar dissociative abilities, the older sister did not develop multiple personality disorder. Why? The answer is probably that her sister (who was four years older than the patient) had developed far more mature nondissociative intrapsychic defenses prior to their mother's death, and did not share the patient's intense sense of disruption.

The precipitating event in this case was the mother's sudden and unexpected death from pneumonia when the patient was seven years old. Three days before she died, the mother had made a special effort to celebrate the patient's first Holy Communion. Although her mother had the symptoms of a cold, she took the patient into Chicago by trolley to buy her a Communion dress. The next day, the mother was too sick to attend either the Communion or the party. On the following day, the patient and her sister came home for lunch, only to see their mother being carried out on a stretcher to a waiting ambulance. The mother died in the hospital the next day.

The mother's death precipitated a hysterical reaction on the part of the surviving members of the family. During this traumatic period, no one paid attention to the patient, who dissociated from this painful series of events and denied the death of her mother. This resulted in a "splitting" of her personality. One part of the patient never mourned the loss of her mother and was constantly awaiting her return. Another part of her attended the funeral and panicked because she thought her mother was going to pull her into the grave. This yielded another split.

The perpetuating phenomena in this case were multifaceted. First, the patient's father had difficulty accepting his wife's death, and subsequently became an alcoholic. He fell at work and developed a hip injury. He was often absent and the excuse was made that he was in the hospital for this injury. Every time the father would come back, he would promise never to leave, but he always did. He kept trying to tell the children that everything was going to be all right; but his conduct clearly indicated that everything was not all right.

During the period following her mother's death, the patient and her sisters went to live with their paternal aunt and uncle. She felt like an outsider in this family, and was semi-ostracized. The patient felt that she was seen as a burden, and was often made the scapegoat. Furthermore, she was very embarrassed on several occasions when her father appeared, flagrantly intoxicated. With no supportive environment available, a steadily increasing sense of anger with the father's behavior fomented yet another "split" in her personality. The new personality "killed" the father at age 13 by denying his existence (for example, "I don't have a father").

Subsequently, this patient developed a social personality in order to cope with school. Another personality was created that dated and eventually married her current husband. The different personalities held the compartmentalized emotions of anger and sadness and were functionally separate from the host.

An interesting parallel in this case that highlights the influence of the family history concerns the fact that the patient's mother was 48 years of age when she died. A year before the patient turned 48, she started to decompensate. She expected to die when she reached this age. This factor underscores the importance of the initial precipitating event and its continued influence on the patient's behavior.

A noteworthy facet of this case is that there was no documented history of abuse. Rather, the mother's sudden and unexpected death triggered the initial split. The development of alternate personalities proceeded as the patient began to dissociate in the face of a repeatedly inconsistent message of love/neglect from both her father and her aunt and uncle. One can see that the model provides a useful clinical framework for understanding this case.

Case Example 2

The second case is a 17-year-old female who was originally seen (by R.G.S.) in the context of family therapy with the mother absent. Her mother and father had recently divorced. The family was in therapy for eight months when treatment was interrupted for logistical reasons. Years later, the therapist learned that the patient had been emotionally and physically abused for her revelations during the family therapy sessions.

After treatment was discontinued, the patient called the therapist and expressed an interest in entering individual psychotherapy. Unfortunately, at that time she could not afford to pay for therapy; a year went by before she got a job and reestablished treatment. Another year went by before the diagnosis of multiple personality disorder was made and confirmed by an independent psychiatrist.

This is not unusual in multiple personality disorder cases. Putnam and colleagues have found that 100 multiple personality disorder patients seen in therapy had been misdiagnosed for an average period of 6.8 years (42).

The individual predisposing factor in this case was the patient's inborn biological capacity to dissociate. Her mother also suffers multiple personality disorder. The family predisposing factors were:

1. The father left the care of the children to the multiple personality disorder mother;

2. The family was large (there were five children) and they did not have enough money for food or clothing;

3. The patient was forced to adopt the role of caretaker because the mother could not function;

4. The father wanted a son and made the patient act like a boy;

5. Family discipline was inconsistent (for example, the patient would be punished for sitting at the table one day, and would not be punished for the same behavior on another day);

6. Family discipline was bizarre (for example, the children were

forced to sit at the table in a military-like manner and were not allowed to leave until all the food was eaten, even if it took eight hours);

7. Three of the siblings were constantly expressing their impulses in both physical and verbal excesses, while the patient and her youngest sister held their emotions in check and were victims of the others' actions;

8. The patient had the burden of intervening in the intersibling abuse;

9. The other children were neglected (for example, the patient and other children were left in their cribs unattended for hours);

10. The family moved five times during the patient's first 12 years of life;

11. The patient attended six different schools, and her social network was continually changing;

12. The family later moved to an ethnic neighborhood where the children were terrorized constantly because they were the only "outsiders."

The precipitating event in this particular case was an abusive, life-threatening experience in which the patient's mother tried to drown her in the bathtub. This incident was later followed by a near-drowning accident at a family picnic. The patient had been left unattended near the water.

Other precipitating events included the patient taking the blame for letting her younger sister (whom she was supposed to be watching) run in front of an oncoming car. Her father's bizarre disciplinary techniques also began to trigger additional splits. For example, when something went wrong, the father would have all the children stand in front of him with their hands facing out. The father would then burn each child's hand until one admitted to the wrongdoing, or he came to believe that they were innocent. The patient reported that her brother was especially resistant to this technique, and once his hands "caught fire." She fearfully added that "burning flesh smells horrible."

The patient, along with her siblings, was also repeatedly starved, and this, too, caused additional breaks. These splits developed into personalities whose adaptive functions fell into five broad categories: 1) intelligence; 2) happiness; 3) sadness; 4) sex; and 5) anger. These five categories also coincided in onset with the five times that the family moved when the patient was a child.

The perpetuating factors in this case were chronic and inconsistent abuse, which continued until the patient moved out of the family home. The family's relocations also served as a perpetuating factor, along with a history of unclear and incongruent parental messages.

Another perpetuating variable in this case was the patient's defensively distorted auditory and visual perception. The family's fighting was heard at an intolerable noise level, and the patient had to dissociate in order to get away from it. She visually distanced herself from her aggressors (both parents and siblings) by perceiving them as if through a telescope, backwards. She would look at her parents shouting at her, and block out the sound of what they were saying. This distorted perception perpetuated the development of separate personalities.

The patient has now been in individual therapy for eight years (seven years since the multiple personality disorder diagnosis). She is currently working on her integration and has continued to make progress. She has managed to leave home and get a responsible job (which she has maintained for eight years). She became able to date, and has married.

This case is an excellent example of how an individual with an inborn capacity to dissociate does so when exposed to repeated, overwhelming anxiety. The patient has continued to be both self-supporting and highly functional. This highlights the adaptive nature of multiple personality disorder. In addition, the proposed model presented in Figure 1 facilitates an ideographic understanding of the dynamics involved in this particular case.

SUMMARY

In the preceding discussion, the authors have described the phenomenon of multiple personality disorder as a genuine diagnostic entity, and have offered a general, nonmathematical model for understanding its development. This model evolved from the authors' collective observations of more than 100 multiple personality disorder cases, and is compatible with the four factor theory of multiple personality disorder recently proposed by Kluft (36). The present model emphasizes that multiple personality disorder only occurs in individuals who have a natural inborn capacity to dissociate, and are exposed to some type of overwhelming anxiety that promotes the continued use of a dissociative defense system. Both predisposing factors are necessary to the development of multiple personality disorder. Neither one alone is sufficient.

The model also recognizes that different precipitating events can cause different dissociative splits. When such events are related by a common adaptational theme, the dissociated elements begin to take on a life history of their own, and an alternate personality begins to develop. Dissociative fragments produced by precipitating events that are not united by a common theme are still present in the system, but do not usually develop into distinct personalities.

The phenomena that perpetuate the multiple personality disorder symptom complex are usually multifaceted. This is because the perpetuating events must be incorporated into and managed within an existing structure of personalities. This structure can be identified by various adaptational themes. In addition, a personality that has developed through a general adaptational theme can be further split into other personalities with more specific adaptive functions. These new personalities then become subsets of the general theme and are not as well developed as the original personality from which they were "cloned."

The heuristic value of the model developed in this discussion stems from its utility as a general descriptive format for the commonalities observed among many multiple personality disorder cases. The authors know of no reported and independently confirmed case of multiple personality disorder that could not be appropriately described by this model. In addition, this model of multiple personality disorder is also clinically useful, in that it also permits an ideographic approach to understanding individual cases. Both considerations are important, because successful treatment is based on a thorough understanding of both the discriminating characteristics of the disorder, and the unique dynamics and contributions of the individual, the family, and society. We hope that this conceptualization will promote a richer understanding of multiple personality disorder.

References

1. Thigpen C, Cleckley H: The Three Faces of Eve. New York, McGraw-Hill, 1957

2. Schreiber FR: Sybil. New York, Henry Regenry, 1973

3. American Psychiatric Association: Diagnostic and Statistical Manual of Mental Disorders (Third Edition). Washington, DC, American Psychiatric Association, 1980

4. Bliss EL: Multiple personalities. Arch Gen Psychiatry 37:1388-1397, 1980

5. Ellenberger HF: The Discovery of the Unconscious. New York, Basic Books, 1980

6. Janet P: L'Automatisme Psychologique. Paris, Felix Alcan, 1889

7. Prince M: The Dissociation of a Personality. New York, Longmans Green, 1906

8. Rosenbaum M: The role of the term schizophrenia in the decline of the diagnosis of multiple personality. Arch Gen Psychiatry 37:1383-1385, 1980

9. Laramore K, Ludwig A, Cain R: Multiple personality: an objective case study. Br J Psychiatry 131:35-40, 1977

10. Braun, BG: Hypnosis creates multiple personality: myth or reality? Int J Clin Exp Hypn 32:191-197, 1984

11. Kluft RP: Varieties of hypnotic interventions in the treatment of multiple personality. Am J Clin Hypn 24:230-240, 1982

12. Kluft RP: An introduction to multiple personality. Psychiatric Annals 14:19-24, 1984

13. Hilgard ER: Divided Consciousness: Multiple Controls in Human Thought and Action. New York, John Wiley and Sons, 1977

14. Bliss EL: Spontaneous self-hypnosis in multiple personality disorder. Psychiatr Clin North Am 7:135-148, 1984

15. Spiegel H, Spiegel D: Trance and treatment. New York, Basic Books, 1978

16. Bower GH: Mood and memory. American Psychologist 36:129-148, 1981

17. Braun BG: Towards a theory of multiple personality and other dissociative phenomena. Psychiatric Clinics of North America 7:171-193, 1984

18. Bliss EL: Multiple personalities, related disorders, and hypnosis. American Journal of Clinical Hypnosis 26:114-123, 1983

19. Lipman LS, Braun BG, Frischholz EJ: Hypnotizability and multiple personality disorder. Paper presented at the First International Conference on Multiple Personality/Dissociative States, Chicago, September, 1984

20. Braun BG: Hypnosis for the diagnosis of multiple personality. Paper presented at a course at the Annual Meeting of the American Psychiatric Association, Chicago, May, 1979

21. Braun BG: Hypnosis for multiple personalities. In Wain HJ (ed.): Clinical Hypnosis in Medicine. Chicago, Year Book Publishers, 1981

22. Caul D: Hypnotherapy in the treatment of multiple personality. Paper presented at the Annual Meeting of the American Psychiatric Association, Atlanta, May, 1978

23. Silberman EK: Memory and dissociation in multiple personalities. Paper presented at the Annual Meeting of the American Psychiatric Association, Los Angeles, May, 1984

24. Morgan AH: The heritability of hypnotic susceptibility in twins. J Abnorm Psychol 82:55-61, 1973

25. Barber TX: Hypnosis: A Scientific Approach. New York, Psychological Dimensions, Inc., 1976

26. Hull CL: Hypnosis and Suggestibility: An Experimental Approach. New York, Appleton-Century, 1933

27. Messerschmidt R: A quantitative investigation of the alleged independent operation of conscious and subconscious process. Journal of Abnormal and Social Psychology 22:325-340, 1927

28. Spanos NP, Barber TX: Toward a convergence in hypnosis research. American Psychologist 29:500-511, 1974

29. White RW, Shevack BJ: Hypnosis and the concept of dissociation. J Abnorm Psychol 37:309-328, 1942

30. Taylor WS, Martin MF: Multiple personality. Journal of Abnormal and Social Psychology 49:281-290, 1944

31. Garcia J: The logic and limits of mental aptitude testing. American Psychologist 36:1172-1180, 1981

32. Matarazzo JD: Wechsler's Measurement and Appraisal of Adult Intelligence, 5th ed. Baltimore, Williams and Wilkins, 1972

33. Sachs RG, Goodwin J, Braun BG: The role of child abuse in the

development of multiple personality disorder, in Multiple Personality and Dissociation. Edited by Braun BG, Kluft RP. New York, Guilford Press (in press)

34. Braun BG: The role of the family in the development of multiple personality disorder. International Journal of Family Psychiatry (in press)

35. Justice B, Justice R: The abusing family. New York, Human Sciences Press, 1976

36. Kluft RP: Treatment of multiple personality disorder. Psychiatr Clin North Am 7:9-30, 1984

37. Allison RB: Psychotherapy of multiple personality. Davis, California, private publication, 1978

38. Fagan J, McMahon PP: Incipient multiple personality in children. J Nerv Ment Dis 172:26-36, 1984

39. Kluft RP: Multiple personality in childhood. Psychiatr Clin North Am 7:121-134, 1984

40. Putnam FW: Childhood multiple personality disorder proposal. Unpublished data, 1981. Reprinted with the author's permission in Kluft RP: Multiple personality in childhood. Psychiatr Clin North Am 7:128

41. Fisher B, Sachs R: A Meta System Model of Child Abuse. Jonesboro, Il, Pilgrimage, 1981

42. Bandura A: The self-system in reciprocal determinism. American Psychologist 33:344-358, 1977

43. Weitzenhoffer AM, Hilgard ER: Stanford Hypnotic Susceptibility Scale, Form C. Palo Alto, Consulting Psychologists Press, 1962

44. Putnam FW, Post RM, Guroff JJ, et al: 100 cases of multiple personality disorder. Presented at the Annual Meeting of the American Psychiatric Association, New Research Abstract #77, New York, May, 1983

4

Dissociation as a Response to Extreme Trauma

Frank W. Putnam, Jr., M.D.

4

Dissociation as a Response to Extreme Trauma

There is an increasing recognition both of the prevalence of chronic dissociative conditions such as multiple personality disorder (1, 2) and of the role of dissociative phenomena in other forms of psychiatric illness (3). This chapter reviews the dissociative disorders recognized by the Diagnostic and Statistical Manual of Mental Disorders, Third Edition (DSM-III), and reviews allied disorders described in the clinical literature. This chapter also examines the relationship between the dissociative process and environmental stress. Variables such as age, gender, concurrent psychiatric diagnosis, and type of trauma will be considered to determine whether they influence the form or course of dissociative reactions.

Dissociation can be defined as a complex psychophysiological process, with psychodynamic triggers, that produces an alteration in the person's consciousness. During this process, thoughts, feelings, and experiences are not integrated into the individual's awareness or memory in the normal way (4-6). Two characteristic features are found in most major dissociative reactions (7). The first is a disturbance in the individual's sense of self-identity. This may take several forms, such as the loss of all self-referential memory in psychogenic amnesia, or the existence of several alternating identities, as is the case with multiple personality disorder. The second feature is a disturbance in the individual's memory that is usually manifested by amnesia for past events or complex acts.

The DSM-III recognizes five categories of dissociative reactions: psychogenic amnesia, psychogenic fugue, multiple personality disorder, depersonalization disorder, and atypical dissociative disorder (8). In clinical practice, these DSM-III distinctions may not always be clear-cut. Features from several DSM-III categories may be present within a patient, either simultaneously or sequentially. It is important to bear in mind that most of the clinical literature on dissociation predates the DSM-III diagnostic criteria. Therefore, discussions of these syndromes in the literature almost inevitably include some cases that could not meet full DSM-III syndromal criteria.

DSM-III DISSOCIATIVE DISORDERS

Psychogenic Amnesia

Psychogenic amnesia is manifested by a " . . . sudden inability to recall important personal information that is too extensive to be explained by ordinary forgetfulness" (8). It is important to rule out memory disturbances caused by an organic mental disorder such as epilepsy or drug intoxication. There are no accurate statistics on the incidence or prevalence of any of the dissociative disorders. However, psychogenic amnesia has been reported to be the most common type of dissociative reaction seen in hospital emergency wards (7). Abeles and Schilder reported that patients presenting with a loss of personal identity accounted for 0.26 percent of new cases admitted to Bellevue psychiatric services in 1934 (9). The incidence of psychogenic amnesia increases significantly in wartime and during natural disasters (8).

Typically, these patients arrive in an emergency room after their confused behavior has brought them to the attention of the authorities. Cases of psychogenic amnesia have been classified into four clinical subtypes, based on the nature of the disturbance in the patients' recall (7, 8). The most commonly described subtype is localized, in which "there is a failure to recall all events occurring during a circumscribed period of time" (8). In selective psychogenic amnesia there is an inability to recall some, but not all, events occurring during a circumscribed period. Less common are generalized amnesia, in which the individual is unable to recall any details of his or her whole life; and continuous amnesia, in which the disturbance in recall is ongoing and encompasses the present moment (8).

The onset of an episode of psychogenic amnesia is usually sudden, and recovery is frequently spontaneous (8, 9). The duration of the episode typically lasts from hours to days, but in rare instances it may extend for up to one month (9–11). Abeles and Schilder reported that 24 percent of their cases have had at least one previous amnestic episode (9). Some authors have reported that sodium amytal has proven more effective for the recovery of information than has hypnosis (10, 12); but other authors maintain that both are equipotent therapeutic techniques (13).

Psychogenic Fugue

Psychogenic fugue is a dissociative reaction manifested by " . . . a sudden, unexpected travel away from home or customary work locale with assumption of a new identity (partial or complete) and an inability to recall one's previous identity" (8). This behavior must occur in the absence of an organic mental disorder. There are no data on the incidence or prevalence of fugue states. While some authors believe that fugue states are rare (14), others state that "there are few psychiatrists who have not met many examples" (15). Despite this divergence of opinion, it is generally reported that the incidence of fugue states increases during times of war, great and generalized civil stress, or natural disasters.

Fugue-like states can occur in a variety of neurological, psychiatric, and toxic conditions. Therefore, the history of fugue is not always indicative of a primary dissociative disorder (16, 17). In the past, some authors divided psychogenic fugue into subgroups, based on the type of amnesia the patient displayed, and the presence or absence of a secondary identity (18, 19). These distinctions do not seem to be useful and have been largely abandoned in the current literature.

There is disagreement over what type of secondary identity is typically elaborated in the fugue state. The DSM-III stresses that this new secondary identity is usually manifested by " . . . more gregarious and uninhibited traits than characterized the former personality, which typically is quiet and altogether ordinary" (8). Other authors, however, have emphasized that the secondary identity has a quiet and prosaic nature, which does not draw attention to itself (7, 20).

Depersonalization Disorder

The experience of depersonalization involves an alteration in the perception of the self so that the individual's sense of reality is lost or altered. This may include feelings of self-estrangement or unreality. There may be alterations in bodily perceptions, such as the sense of becoming very large or small; or the feeling that one's bodily parts do not belong to one; or the feeling that one's bodily parts have changed in size. The individual may have out-of-body experiences in which the person views himself or herself as if from a distance or from above. The person may report feeling "dead," "mechanical," or as if "in a dream."

Depersonalization in and of itself is a very common phenomenon. Thirty to 70 percent of young adults experience mild forms of depersonalization (8, 21). Even Freud has described his own experience of depersonalization (22, 23). Cattell has noted that in psychiatric patients, symptoms of depersonalization are the third most common group of complaints, following depression and anxiety in frequency (24). In most patients the symptoms appear suddenly but remit much more slowly. Only about 10 percent of cases report severe or lasting experiences. Dizziness or episodes of fainting are frequently associated with experiences of depersonalization (7). Derealization, a feeling of unreality or detachment from the environment, is usually present, in addition to feelings of depersonalization.

Depersonalization is considered a psychiatric disorder of clinical significance when there are " . . . one or more episodes of depersonalization that are sufficient to produce significant impairment in social or occupational functioning" (8). This must be due to primary depersonalization and not a result of depersonalization secondary to another psychiatric condition, such as schizophrenia, anxiety disorder, epilepsy, affective disorders, or an organic mental disorder.

Multiple Personality Disorder

Multiple personality disorder can be understood as a chronic or persistent dissociative reaction. This syndrome has been described since the 1700s. In all likelihood, many of the cases of demonic possession seen in earlier times were instances of this disorder, being both experienced by its victims and understood by its interpreters as the incursion of evil entities (25). Subsequently, clinicians working with these patients have offered a number of definitions and diagnostic criteria for the disorder (26–29), but the first formalized and generally accepted diagnostic criteria were not established until the publication of the DSM-III. These criteria require: "The existence within the individual of two or more distinct personalities, each of which is dominant at a particular time. The personality that is dominant at any particular time determines the individual's behavior. Each individual personality is complex and integrated with its own unique behavior patterns and social relationships" (8).

The incidence and prevalence of this disorder is unknown. The number of case reports and references to multiple personality disorder in the clinical literature has shown a remarkable waxing and waning over the years. During the period from 1880 to 1910, there were numerous articles and books on the subject and a general public fascination with the phenomena expressed in personal accounts and novels (30, 31). This expressed interest fell to an all-time low during the 1960s but has skyrocketed in the last decade, with over 150 recent clinical articles and books on the subject, and hundreds of accounts in the media. The reasons for this cyclic waxing and waning of recognized cases are not clear, but may include fluctuations in the popularity of hypnosis as a diagnostic and therapeutic tool, a skeptical or negative reaction to the claims and allegations made by early investigators of multiple personality disorder (31), and the rise of schizophrenia as a diagnostic entity (32). Currently, over 1,000 contemporary cases have been identified in North America, and many investigators believe that this is the tip of the iceberg (33).

The earliest descriptions of this disorder were primarily single case reports. However, in the last few years, a number of case collections have been published, allowing further characterization of multiple personality disorder (3, 25, 34-36). Most multiple personality disorder patients have been misdiagnosed as having depression, borderline or sociopathic personality disorder, or schizophrenia. Putnam studied a series of 100 cases and found the average number of personalities per patient was 13.3 (36). The average was 13.9 in a series reported by Kluft, who described 33 patients who had been integrated for a minimum of 27 months (34).

The personalities described by clinicians working with multiple personality disorder patients usually include a number of frequently encountered types of alternate personalities, which perform specific functions or roles in the individual's life. These alternates commonly include: child personalities, who may serve to hold or buffer traumatic experiences; persecutor personalities, who inflict pain and punishment on the individual (often through suicide attempts or self-mutilation); helper personalities, who provide advice or perform functions that the host or central personality is unable to accomplish; and recorder or memory personalities, who maintain continuous awareness in spite of the amnesias experienced by other personalities. In addition, there may be personalities who perceive themselves as being of the opposite sex, or having opinions and life-styles that are in dramatic opposition to that of the host or main personality (34, 36).

Atypical Dissociative Disorder

Atypical dissociative disorder is a final catch-all category established by the DSM-III to include "... those individuals who appear to have a dissociative disorder but do not satisfy the criteria for a specific dissociative disorder. Examples include trance-like states, derealization unaccompanied by depersonalization, and those more prolonged dissociated states that may occur in persons who have been subjected to periods of prolonged and intense coercive persuasion (brainwashings, thought reform, and indoctrination while the captive of terrorists or cultists)" (8). The creation of this residual category acknowledges the clinical fact that many examples of dissociation do not neatly fall into one of the above syndromes, but are sufficiently disabling to be classified as a psychiatric disorder.

THE LINKAGE OF DISSOCIATION TO EXTREME STRESS

The Wartime Amnesic Syndromes

The wartime amnesic syndromes are a group of dissociative reactions, primarily psychogenic amnesias and psychogenic fugue states, that are observed in soldiers and civilians during war. Amnesia is fairly common in wartime; five to 20 percent of veterans report amnesia for their combat experiences (37, 38). Other manifestations of dissociative processes associated with wartime experiences include persistent feelings of detachment, estrangement, and flashbacks, which constitute part of the post-traumatic stress disorder frequently reported in combat veterans (39).

Estimates of the incidence of amnesic syndromes in war range from five to 14 percent of all psychiatric casualties (37, 40–43). The precipitants of these dissociative reactions are often "terror, bomb blast, or exhaustion" (37, 40). A high incidence of head injury or loss of consciousness, however, has been reported in this population, and may well contribute an organic element to the amnesia (37). There does seem to be a direct relationship between the incidence of amnesia and the degree of stress experienced by the individual (37, 40). Sargent and Slater ordered their cases into three groups by the degree of stress experienced by the patient. Soldiers in the severe stress group, who had experienced prolonged marching and fighting under heavy enemy fire, had a 35 percent incidence of amnesic syndromes. Soldiers who only experienced periodic bombings or fighting sustained a 13 percent incidence of amnesic symptoms. Those exposed only to the normal life of a base camp without combat exposure suffered a six percent incidence of amnesia (40). In contrast, Kirshner reported an overall incidence of 1.3 percent for dissociative reactions in a peacetime military setting (44).

The existence of a predisposing constitutional factor has been stressed by some authors as important in the psychogenesis of wartime amnesias. Sargent and Slater noted that a "constitutional inferiority" was particularly prominent in those patients who had amnesic episodes in the absence of combat stress. Approximately 88 percent of this group suffered fugue episodes (40). Henderson and Moore found that 71 percent of their cases came from home situations judged by the authors to be moderately to severely disturbed. They offer the opinion that " ... this is the most important of all the predisposing factors that have been analyzed" (37).

Peacetime Amnesic Syndromes

The role of acute trauma in precipitating psychogenic amnesias has also been noted in several peacetime case collections. Abeles and Schilder reported that "Some unpleasant conflict, either financial or familial, was significant in the immediate cause of the amnesia" (9). Kanzer felt that he could establish that acute emotional problems were involved in the etiology of 59 percent of his sample of amnesic patients. He noted that "Where acute disturbances were lacking, the primary etiological agent sometimes appeared to be other than psychogenic ... " (10). Kiersch, however, found that only 25 percent of his sample of psychogenic amnesia cases were dealing with "severe reality factors" (12).

Three general categories of precipitant experiences associated with psychogenic fugue have been identified by reviewers of this syndrome. The first is a situation in which the individual can neither fight nor escape an anticipated danger (14, 18, 19, 45). The second commonly observed precipitant is the threatened or actual loss of an important object (46, 47). The third precipitant is an overwhelming, panic-inspiring impulse, such as a homicidal or suicidal urge (18, 48, 49).

Investigators of psychogenic fugue disagree on the temporal linkage of these precipitant factors to the actual onset of the fugue episode. Berrington et al. stress the immediate nature of the precipitant in cases in which the individual is escaping from an intolerable situation. They found evidence for such an immediate precipitant in 95 percent of their cases (14). Akhtar and Brenner also note a temporal relationship between the onset of fugue and psychological stress (16). In his first analysis of 25 cases of fugue, Stengel states, "Emotional trauma in some cases appear to have closely preceded the first attack" (49). In a subsequent reanalysis of his case data, Stengel revised this assessment to "The fugue with impulse to wander is only very rarely precipitated directly by a preceding overt psychic trauma . . . " (48). This discrepancy may be due to a difference in the sample populations analyzed. Berrington et al. point out that their patients differed from Stengel's significantly on several variables such as head injury, childhood history, and current psychopathology (14).

Those authors who do not find evidence of immediate traumatic precipitants stress the existence of a long-standing psychological disturbance in individuals who experience fugue episodes. Stengel, in particular, emphasizes a history of disturbed child-parent relationships in his cases. He found "Investigations into the individual histories of the patients revealed with surprising consistency serious abnormality in the relations to home life" (49). "The individual case histories of these patients reveal one characteristic feature. They are persons during whose development there has occurred a serious disturbance in the child-parent relation, usually of such a nature that relationship to one or both parents was either completely lacking or only partially developed" (50). Other authors dispute the universality of this finding and note a lower incidence of unhappy childhood or disturbed child-parent relations in their samples (14, 19).

The real or threatened loss of an important object has been identified as a precipitant factor in several psychoanalytic models of psychogenic fugue. Geleerd, Hacker, and Rapaport stress the role of intense separation anxiety and the close relationship of fugue states to sleep (46). Luparello adds the existence of suicidal wishes and murderous impulses to this model (19). The existence of depression and warded-off suicidal impulses in psychogenic fugue states has been commented on by a variety of investigators (18, 19, 46, 48). Homicidal impulses appear to be a factor in a smaller percentage of cases (18).

Depersonalization

Depersonalization is a ubiquitous phenomenon that is found in a wide range of psychiatric and neurologic conditions, including: schizophrenia (52); depression (53); phobic anxiety states (54); obsessive-compulsive disorder (55); drug abuse (56); sleep deprivation (57); temporal lobe epilepsy (58); and migraine headache (59). Depersonalization is also seen in "normal" populations (21, 60–63). The overall incidence of depersonalization ranges from 8.5 percent (63) to 70 percent (61) depending upon the methodology and definitions used in the study. No single etiology, model, or common life experience seems to account for the widespread nature of depersonalization.

The linkage of depersonalization to traumatic experiences is most clearly demonstrated by two lines of evidence. The first is the high incidence of depersonalization noted in survivors of sustained traumatic experiences, such as concentration camps (64–67). Depersonalization was often part of the initial shock reaction of the individual upon being placed in a camp (65, 66) and later became a sustained experience upon release from the camp (64, 68).

The second linkage of depersonalization to trauma comes from the work by Noyes and others on psychological responses to life-threatening danger (69–71). In a series of studies, Noyes and his colleagues have retrospectively examined the experiences of individuals in the face of life-threatening events. They identified the existence of a "transient depersonalization syndrome" that approximately one-third of their subjects experienced during life-threatening episodes (70, 71). They compared the symptoms of this "transient depersonalization syndrome" elicited by near-death experiences with the depersonalization symptoms experienced in a group of hospitalized psychiatric patients, and concluded that the two experiences were largely similar. The authors, however, noted a tendency for depersonalization phenomena associated with life-threatening experiences to lead to an increase in alertness, while the psychiatric patient group associated their depersonalization experiences with a clouding of mental processes.

Hypnoid States

Breuer and Freud, in *Studies on Hysteria*, described the existence of "hypnoid states," which were abnormal states of consciousness associated with a "splitting" of consciousness, or dissociative process. They described these states as " . . . a clearly abnormal mental condition, such as the half-hypnotic twilight state of daydreams, auto-hypnosis, and the like" (72). A number of psychoanalytic studies have suggested that there is a linkage between hypnoid states and early childhood trauma. Fliess sees the hypnoid state as an evasion that protects against the work of remembering earlier trauma (73). Loewald notes the relationship of hypnoid states to "traumatic" experiences, which the immature ego is unable to cope with by abreaction or associative absorption (74). Dickes also comments on the defensive utilization of hypnoid states originating in major childhood trauma (75). Silver provides a graphic account of the association of childhood sexual abuse with hypnoid states in an adult patient (76).

Multiple Personality Disorder

All of the recent reviews and case collections of multiple personality disorder indicate that this syndrome, while usually not diagnosed until adulthood, has its origins in childhood (1, 2, 8, 25). Childhood cases of multiple personality disorder have been diagnosed, and case collections of child and adolescent victims are beginning to appear in the clinical literature (77, 78). The evidence from both the child and adult cases indicates that childhood trauma, particularly sexual and/or physical abuse, is a primary etiologic factor in the genesis of the disorder (1, 2, 25, 36, 79-81)

In the vast majority of recorded cases, the first splitting off of an alternate personality appears to occur within a window of vulnerability extending from age six months to approximately 12 years (2, 25, 36, 81). A few cases are reported in which the appearance of an alternate personality is said to have occurred in late adolescence or early adulthood (25, 36). In most instances, both the first splitting off of an alternate personality and many subsequent splits of alternate personalities occur in the context of immediate overwhelming trauma.

The documentation of trauma is difficult in adult patients, whose retrospective reports are subject to all of the usual distortions of time and memory. In one series of 106 adult multiple personality disorder cases, there was outside verification of childhood trauma in 15 percent of the patients (82). The National Institute of Mental Health (NIMH) child multiple personality disorder identification project has focused exclusively on children coming from situations where child abuse or other trauma is documentable. At the present time, all cases of multiple personality disorder diagnosed in children in this study have had a verifiable history of either child abuse or massive psychic trauma, such as witnessing the massacre of family members. In most cases, the trauma took the form of sexual abuse, usually incest. In addition, several children had histories of physical abuse and/or confinement abuses, such as being locked in closets, cellars, or trunks, being buried alive, or being repeatedly bound and gagged.

The linkage between the development of a dissociative reaction and the experience of overwhelming psychic trauma is most clear-cut in multiple personality disorder. All of the recent case reports, case collections, and surveys indicate that the vast majority of multiple personality patients report histories of childhood trauma. In the NIMH case survey, only three percent of the cases were reported by their therapists as having no evidence of childhood trauma (36). All of those cases were in an early phase of treatment (one year duration or less) and memory for childhood traumatic events may well have been still shielded by amnestic barriers at that point in treatment.

Atypical Dissociative Disorder

Atypical dissociative disorder is linked to extreme stress in the DSM-III definition (8). This category covers transient trance-states, derealization with depersonalization, and prolonged dissociative states seen in persons suffering from extremely stressful experiences such as brainwashing, being held hostage by terrorists, and the like.

FACTORS INFLUENCING THE TYPE OF DISSOCIATIVE REACTION

Age

Mayer-Gross first commented in 1935 on the apparent relationship between age and the frequency of depersonalization symptoms in psychiatric patients. "In spite of the varying degree of severity of the illness I found a striking uniformity of age at the beginning of the syndrome: only six patients were over 30 then, the oldest of these being 39" (83). Later investigators also noted this trend. Shorvon reported that the average age of his patients was 24.5 years for females and 23.5 years for males. "A quarter of the cases had a sudden onset of depersonalization between the ages of 15 and 19" (84). Davison believed that his collection of cases supported the idea that " . . . there exists a primary idiopathic depersonalization which usually starts suddenly in adolescence and often recurs over a period of years" (85). Sedman found that the average age of subjects experiencing depersonalization was 25 years, while his control group of depressed and anxious patients averaged 35 years of age. The results, however, did not reach statistical significance (61). Brauer et al., in a questionnaire study of depersonalization in Yale-New Haven Hospital inpatients, found that "Demographic data indicated strongly that younger

patients have higher depersonalization scores than older patients"
(86). Tucker et al. replicated this finding in a similar study in the
same setting (87). Fleiss et al. found a statistically significant
relationship between age and the presence of depersonalization
symptoms. Younger patients were more likely ($p < .05$) to report
depersonalization than were older patients (88). Parikh et al. have
also found a similar effect, which was significant at the $p < .01$
level (89).

The relationship of age to onset of psychogenic amnesia or
psychogenic fugue episodes is not well delineated. Abeles and
Schilder simply noted that 80 percent of their cases with psychogenic loss of personal identity were in the second, third, or fourth
decade (9). Kanzer found that age distribution for his psychogenic
amnesia cases indicated that most patients were in the third or
fourth decade of life (10). Wilson et al. found no significant
difference with respect to age in his group of amnesic patients (51).
Kirshner's survey of dissociative reactions in the peacetime military found that the dissociators had an average age of 24.5 years,
compared to the control group of other nonalcoholic, psychiatric
admissions, which averaged 27.8 years (44). Kiersch found that the
"majority" of his amnesia patients were in the 21 to 30 age group
(12). Stengel reported an average age of 22.7 years for the onset of a
first psychogenic fugue (49). Berrington et al., however, noted that
their population of fugue patients averaged 31.98 years of age (14).
These data suggest that psychogenic amnesia and psychogenic
fugue states tend to be found in patients under 40 years of age, but
are not as clearly associated with adolescence and early adulthood
as is depersonalization.

An analysis of the case data available for multiple personality
disorder indicates that this syndrome tends to be diagnosed in the
late 20s to early 30s. A review of 38 case reports in the literature,
meeting retrospectively applied DSM-III criteria, found an average
age at diagnosis of 28.5 years. Collections of cases by Bliss and
Allison reported mean ages at diagnosis of 30 years and 29.4 years,
respectively (25, 90). Kluft has reported a mean age of 36.1 years for
his cohort of 33 cases upon completion of treatments averaging
21.6 months (34). A survey of 100 independent cases found a

mean age at diagnosis of 31.3 years (36). Thus, all of the current data indicates that this syndrome is usually not recognized until the third to fourth decade.

The onset of multiple personality disorder, as discussed in the section above, appears to be much earlier. The data at present, although scanty, strongly indicate that the first alternate personalities appear in childhood, usually between the ages of six months and 12 years. Prospective studies currently under way may help to clarify the age range and context in which multiple personality disorder develops.

Gender

A comparison of the female to male ratio in case collections of depersonalization subjects drawn from civilian populations indicates a trend toward more female cases. Several authors report that they found no association of depersonalization with gender (21, 86, 88, 89). All of the remaining group studies contained more women than men. Gittleson (87) and Tucker et al. (91) both report female to male ratios of 1.6:1; and Nuller (92) reports a ratio of 2.6:1. Roberts (60), in his study of depersonalization phenomena in students, found a female to male ratio of 3.0:1; Mayer-Gross (83) reports a ratio of 4.0:1 in his collection of 25 patients.

The data available for the civilian peacetime amnesic syndromes indicates no evidence for linkage to gender. Abeles and Schilder reported a 1:1 ratio, and Kanzer found a 0.73:1 ratio for cases of psychogenic amnesia (9, 10). Stengel's collection of 36 cases of fugue contained 23 females to 13 males (1.76:1), but Berrington et al. noted that Stengel picked most of his patients from the female wards of Bristol Mental Hospital (14, 48, 49). Berrington, however, found a preponderance of male fugue cases with a ratio of 0.19:1 (14).

The case collections of multiple personality disorder all indicate a significant association between gender and the presence of the disorder. The magnitude of this association, however, has declined as more cases are added to the literature. Allison reported an 8:1 female to male ratio for cases that he diagnosed (90). Bliss noted a

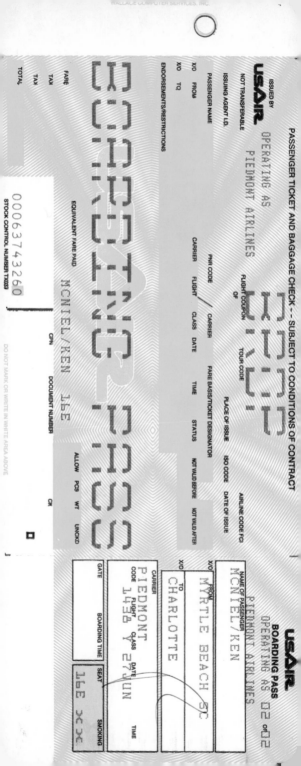

PASSENGER TICKET AND BAGGAGE CHECK -- SUBJECT TO CONDITIONS OF CONTRACT

ISSUED BY USAir
OPERATING AS
PIEDMONT AIRLINES

NOT TRANSFERABLE

ISSUING AGENT I.D.

PASSENGER NAME

X/O FROM

X/O TO

ENDORSEMENTS/RESTRICTIONS

FARE

X/O

X/O

TOTAL$

TAX

TAX

FLIGHT COUPON
OF

PNR CODE

CARRIER   FLIGHT   CARRIER   CLASS   DATE   TIME

TOUR CODE

FARE BASIS/TICKET DESIGNATOR   STATUS

PLACE OF ISSUE

ISO CODE   DATE OF ISSUE

AIRLINE CODE FCI

NOT VALID BEFORE   NOT VALID AFTER

ALLOW   PCS   WT   UNCKD   CK

BOARDING PASS

EQUIVALENT FARE PAID

MCNIEL/KEN   16E

CPN   DOCUMENT NUMBER

STOCK CONTROL NUMBER TX033
0006374326D

DO NOT MARK OR WRITE IN WHITE AREA ABOVE

USAir
BOARDING PASS
OPERATING AS   02 of 02
PIEDMONT AIRLINES

NAME OF PASSENGER
MCNIEL/KEN

X/O FROM
MYRTLE BEACH SC

X/O TO
CHARLOTTE

CARRIER
PIEDMONT
CODE

FLIGHT   CLASS   DATE
1438   Y   27 JUN

GATE   BOARDING TIME   SEAT   SMOKING
16E   X X

TIME

PASSENGER TICKET AND BAGGAGE CHECK

PASSENGER COUPON

NOTICE

SUBJECT TO TARIFF REGULATIONS

(NOT FOR USE IN MAGNETIC STRIPE READERS)

If the passenger's journey involves an ultimate destination or stop in a country other than the country of departure the Warsaw Convention may be applicable and the Convention governs and in most cases limits the liability of carriers for death or personal injury and in respect of loss of or damage to baggage. See also notice headed "Advice to International Passengers on Limitation of Liability."

CONDITIONS OF CONTRACT

1. As used in this contract "ticket" means this passenger ticket and baggage check, of which these conditions and the notices form part, "carriage" is equivalent to "transportation", "carrier" means all air carriers that carry or undertake to carry the passenger or his baggage hereunder or perform any other service incidental to such air carriage. "WARSAW CONVENTION" means the Convention for the Unification of Certain Rules Relating to International Carriage by Air signed at Warsaw, 12th October 1929, or that Convention as amended at The Hague, 28th September 1955, whichever may be applicable.

2. Carriage hereunder is subject to the rules and limitations relating to liability established by the Warsaw Convention unless such carriage is not "international carriage" as defined by that Convention.

3. To the extent not in conflict with the foregoing carriage and other services performed by each carrier are subject to: (I) provisions contained in this ticket, (II) applicable tariffs, (III) carrier's conditions of carriage and related regulations which are made part hereof (and are available on application at the offices of carrier), except in transportation between a place in the United States or Canada and any place outside thereof to which tariffs in force in those countries apply.

4. Carrier's name may be abbreviated in the ticket, the full name and its abbreviation being set forth in carrier's tariffs, conditions of carriage, regulations or timetables; carrier's address shall be the airport of departure shown opposite the first abbreviation of carrier's name in the ticket; the agreed stopping places are those places set forth in this ticket or as shown in carrier's timetables as scheduled stopping places on the passenger's route; carriage to be performed hereunder by several successive carriers is regarded as a single operation.

5. An air carrier issuing a ticket for carriage over the lines of another air carrier does so only as its agent.

6. Any exclusion or limitation of liability of carrier shall apply to and be for the benefit of agents, servants and representatives of carrier and any person whose aircraft is used by carrier for carriage and its agents, servants and representatives.

7. Checked baggage will be delivered to bearer of the baggage check. In case of damage to baggage moving in international transportation complaint must be made in writing to carrier forthwith after discovery of damage and, at the latest, within 7 days from receipt; in case of delay, complaint must be made within 21 days from date the baggage was delivered. See tariffs or conditions of carriage regarding non-international transportation.

8. This ticket is good for carriage for one year from date of issue, except as otherwise provided in this ticket, in carrier's tariffs, conditions of carriage, or related regulations. The fare for carriage hereunder is subject to change prior to commencement of carriage. Carrier may refuse transportation if the applicable fare has not been paid.

9. Carrier undertakes to use its best efforts to carry the passenger and baggage with reasonable dispatch. Times shown in timetable or elsewhere are not guaranteed and form no part of this contract. Carrier may without notice substitute alternate carriers or aircraft, and may alter or omit stopping places shown on the ticket in case of necessity. Schedules are subject to change without notice. Carrier assumes no responsibility for making connections.

10. Passenger shall comply with Government travel requirements, present exit, entry and other required documents and arrive at airport by time fixed by carrier or, if no time is fixed, early enough to complete departure procedures.

11. No agent, servant or representative of carrier has authority to alter, modify or waive any provision of this contract unless authorized by a corporate officer of carrier.

female to male ratio of greater than 14:1 (25), and Putnam et al. found a ratio of 9:1 in 100 cases independently reported by therapists (36). Recently, Stern has reported a 7:1 sex ratio, while three experienced therapists have found much lower sex ratios of 4:1, 2.6:1, and 2.18:1 (35, 81, 93, 94).

Several authors have indicated that a significant sampling bias probably exists in all of the recently published case collections of multiple personality disorder (1, 2, 95). It is felt that, due to the prevalence of violence in this disorder, many male victims of multiple personality disorder are probably resident in the criminal justice system and are therefore under-represented in patient samples. Female multiple personality disorder victims, whose violence tends to be more self-directed, are more likely to be seen in the mental health system. The single published study of the incidence of multiple personality disorder in a criminal population indicated that 13 out of 33 sexual offenders had multiple personality disorder (3).

Concurrent Diagnosis

Depersonalization is found across a wide range of psychiatric and neurologic diagnoses. These conditions include psychotic and nonpsychotic forms of psychiatric illness, and both temporal lobe and other forms of epilepsy, migraine syndromes, accidents, and traumatic situations, as well as the abuse of certain psychoactive drugs. Fleiss found that the 15 percent of the 866 hospitalized adult mental patients studied in the United States-United Kingdom diagnostic project had experienced symptoms of depersonalization within the month before admission to the hospital (88).

The psychotic illnesses include schizophrenia and manic-depressive psychoses. Brauer et al. found the overall incidence of schizophrenia to be 30 percent in their collection of patients with depersonalization (86). Tucker et al. noted that 53 percent of their depersonalized patients had "classic schizophrenia" (87). Parikh et al. made the diagnosis of schizophrenia in 66 percent of their depersonalized patients (89). Hwu et al. suggest that the presence of derealization/depersonalization is a favorable prognostic sign in schizophrenic patients (96). The reported incidence of psychotic depression in depersonalized patients ranges from 13 percent to 40 percent (86, 87, 91). Gittleson has shown that the presence of depersonalization symptoms is independent of the presence of delusions in depressive psychosis (91).

The neurotic disorders that are most commonly associated with depersonalization include depression, phobic-anxiety syndromes, and obsessive-compulsive disorder. The incidence of neurotic depression ranges from 15 percent to 32 percent in patients with depersonalization syndromes (86, 87, 89). Oberndorf first popularized the idea of a linkage between depersonalization and anxiety (97). This observation was later expanded by Roth and his co-workers into the phobic anxiety-depersonalization syndrome (54). A strong linkage between obsessional traits and depersonalization has also been reported. Shorvon noted an 88 percent incidence of obsessional symptoms in his case collection of depersonalized patients (84). Roth also found that 74 percent of his patients had strong premorbid obsessional traits (54). Other authors have observed similar findings (55, 61, 98).

Depersonalization is also reported in neurologic disorders, primarily epilepsy and migraine headache. Hughlings Jackson first commented on this (99), and later Penfield and Jasper made systematic observations of this phenomenon in their patients (100). The incidence of depersonalization derealization symptoms in these neurologic populations remains to be quantified.

Noyes has noted a 30 percent incidence of depersonalization syndrome in accident victims (70). Fullerton et al. note a similar phenomenon in spinal cord injury patients, with 60 percent reporting a depersonalization reaction immediately following the accident. Patients with quadriplegia were most likely to experience a depersonalization reaction (101).

Fugue states are also seen in a wide variety of psychiatric and neurologic disorders. These include epileptic fugues with an incidence ranging from 6.4 percent in unspecified epilepsy to 74 percent in temporal lobe epilepsy (16). Other organic etiologies have also been noted, including brain tumor, head trauma, corticosteroid toxicity, hypoglycemia, uremia, and malaria (16).

Fugues are also noted in schizophrenia and depression (14, 16, 48, 49). The frequency of fugue in these psychiatric illnesses is unknown but must be uncommon, as fugue is not included in any diagnostic criteria for these disorders.

Cases of psychogenic amnesia usually do not carry a concurrent psychiatric diagnosis. Both Abeles and Schilder (9) and Kanzer (10) comment on the frequency of depressive symptoms in many of their amnesic patients.

Patients with multiple personality disorder are often misdiagnosed, and have received an average of 3.6 psychiatric or neurologic diagnoses prior to the diagnosis of multiple personality disorder (36). The existence of concurrent psychiatric diagnoses in these patients is difficult to determine because of the dramatic shifts in mood and behavior secondary to alternate personality switches. The diagnosis of multiple personality disorder should be considered the superordinate psychiatric diagnosis, since full syndromal criteria for other disorders are rarely met (95). Some authors have argued that multiple personality disorder is a variant of borderline personality disorder (102). Other authors have found a borderline organization in 15 percent to 70 percent of their cases, but note that not all multiple personality disorder patients meet stringent criteria for borderline personality disorder (34, 35).

The evidence indicates that all of the major dissociative symptoms can occur in the context of a wide variety of psychiatric and neurologic conditions. This suggests that dissociation is a process, similar to paranoia, which cuts across diagnostic categories.

Type of Trauma

In a review of this type it is impossible to quantify the severity of the traumata reported in connection with case descriptions of dissociative reactions noted in the clinical literature. However, it was feasible to catalog the types of trauma described in association with each type of dissociative disorder, to see if any patterns emerged. An attempt was made to determine whether there was evidence for the hypothesis that specific types of trauma influenced the form of the dissociative reaction.

In the case of the wartime amnesic syndromes, the precipitating trauma was primarily combat-related and involved either direct physical threats to the individual, or the witnessing of the violent death of friends. In some cases, secondary fugues occurred when the individual was reconfronted with memories of the original fugue-invoking event through experiences such as seeing a war movie. The same types of amnesic syndromes, however, were reported to occur in peacetime, where the precipitating trauma was often the loss of a loved one, a financial reverse, or difficulties in an important relationship.

Thus, at this level of comparison, the specific type of trauma does not seem to influence the precipitation of psychogenic amnesia or psychogenic fugue reactions. The symptoms of depersonalization also seem to occur within a wide range of contexts, from "idiopathic" depersonalization without an obvious precipitant, to depersonalization syndromes accompanying life-threatening danger and severe physical injury. In multiple personality disorder there is evidence that sexual abuse, particularly incest, seems to be involved in the majority of cases (1, 2, 25, 36, 79–81). Other forms of abuse, both physical and emotional, may also be reported in these cases, so that no clear argument can be made for specificity of sexual abuse to multiple personality disorder at present. With the possible exception of multiple personality disorder, the type of traumatic event experienced by the individual does not seem to influence the specific form of dissociative reaction.

ARE CHILDREN MORE PRONE TO DISSOCIATIVE REACTIONS THAN ADULTS?

A number of lines of circumstantial evidence suggest that children may be more prone than adults to use dissociation as a defensive mechanism for coping with stress. Reports of dissociative reactions in children are rare compared to reports of dissociative reactions in adults (103). Many adult patients with depersonalization, however, report that their first episode occurred in childhood. The experiential descriptions of children with depersonalization syndromes are essentially the same as those reported by adults (104). The tendency of depersonalization to occur more frequently in younger persons suggests that these symptoms may be more common in children than is usually recognized.

The capacity to be hypnotized may be directly related to a propensity to utilize a dissociative mechanism for coping with trauma (3, 34, 94, 105). Several studies have suggested that children are more hypnotizable than are adults (106–108). In general, both longitudinal and cross-sectional studies indicate that children show an increasing responsiveness to hypnosis from the age of five to about the age of 10 to 14 years. This is followed by a decline during adolescence to an adult level (109–111). Gardiner has suggested that children under the age of five may be excellent hypnotic subjects if the appropriate induction and scaling techniques are applied (112). If hypnotizability is associated with an increased utilization of dissociative mechanisms for coping with trauma, then children, with their greater hypnotizability, may be more likely to invoke dissociative defenses.

A secondary line of evidence bearing on this thesis is the finding that one of the best correlates of hypnotizability in adults is a childhood history of severe punishment (113–115). Hilgard has suggested that children subject to strict discipline and punishment cultivate fantasy as an escape, which predisposes them to high hypnotic susceptibility.

Imaginary companionship, a normal childhood developmental phenomenon, may also provide a nidus for the development of alternate personalities in multiple personality disorder (94). Svendsen has defined imaginary companionship as " . . . an invisible character, named and referred to in conversation with other persons or played with directly for a period of time, . . . having an air of reality for the child but no apparent objective basis" (116). Different authors have reported an incidence of imaginary companionship in children ranging from 13 percent to 65 percent, depending upon the age group surveyed and the definitional criteria employed (116, 117).

The origins and functions of imaginary companions appear to

be diverse, but many authors note that prelatency children create imaginary companions when faced with neglect or hostility. These companions then often provide an organizing scheme in memory that subsumes earlier traumata (119). Myers has reported on several adult patients experiencing depersonalization phenomena who reactivated the imaginary companions associated with earlier traumata during the course of psychoanalysis (119). One of the many functions of imaginary companionship is to support the child in situations where he or she feels frightened or lonely. Children who suffer prolonged or repetitive abuse or trauma may come to depend on the support and companionship of these imaginary constructs, which perhaps become transformed into alternate personalities over time.

SUMMARY

A review of the clinical literature pertinent to the DSM-III dissociative disorders indicates that in most patients the precipitation of a dissociative reaction is associated with substantial psychological stress or traumatic experiences. The incidence and prevalence of the dissociative disorders is unknown. Multiple personality disorder, however, is becoming increasingly recognized, and the number of cases reported in the literature now exceeds those for psychogenic amnesia and psychogenic fugue states. In times of war or generalized stress, the overall incidence of dissociative reactions appears to rise significantly.

Factors that appear to be associated with a vulnerability to dissociative reactions include age, gender, and a history of a disturbed childhood. Dissociative reactions in general are more likely to occur in individuals below the age of 40, and depersonalization in particular is significantly more frequent in adolescents and young adults. Multiple personality disorder appears to originate in childhood, but is generally not diagnosed until adulthood. Gender appears to be linked to depersonalization disorder and to multiple personality disorder, but this apparent connection should be viewed with caution, as it may reflect a substantial bias in case sampling. A childhood history of a disturbed home situation has been noted as a significant factor predisposing the individual to psychogenic amnesia or psychogenic fugue states in both wartime and peacetime contexts. In multiple personality disorder, a childhood history of severe sexual and/or physical abuse has been reported in the vast majority of cases. Children may be more prone to use dissociative defenses for coping with trauma than adults, due to their higher hypnotic susceptibility and the existence of normal developmental phenomena, such as imaginary companions and other fantasy equivalents that may be used as coping mechanisms in times of stress.

Concurrent psychiatric diagnosis does not appear to be linked directly to the presence of dissociative symptoms. There is a 15 percent to 20 percent incidence of dissociative symptoms in psychiatric patients, irrespective of diagnosis. Dissociation, in its varying manifestations, appears to be a process, like paranoia or hallucinations, that can occur in psychiatric, neurologic, medical, and toxic conditions.

While the current data are very scanty, multiple personality disorder appears to be unique among the dissociative disorders in that without treatment, it is a chronic condition compared to the generally self-limited course of the other dissociative reactions. Multiple personality disorder also appears to occur in the relatively specific context of an age range from infancy to early adolescence, and in persons with a history of repetitive sexual and/or physical abuse. More research is required to determine whether this apparent specificity of developmental vulnerability and abuse history is, in fact, significant in the etiology of multiple personality disorder.

References

1. Boor M: The multiple personality epidemic: additional cases and inferences regarding diagnosis, etiology, dynamics and treatment. J Nerv Ment Dis 170:302-304, 1982

2. Greaves GB: Multiple personality 165 years after Mary Reynolds. J Nerv Ment Dis 168:577-597, 1980

3. Bliss EL: Multiple personalities, related disorders and hypnosis. Am J Clin Hypn 26:114-123, 1983

4. West LJ: Dissociative reaction, in Comprehensive Textbook of Psychiatry, 2nd ed. Edited by Freedman AM, Kaplan HI. Baltimore, Williams and Wilkins, 1967

5. Kluft RP: The psychophysiology of multiple personality disorder: analytic perspectives. Paper presented at the American Psychiatric Association Annual Meeting, Los Angeles, May, 1984

6. Putnam FW: Diagnosing multiple personality disorder. Medical Aspects of Human Sexuality (in press)

7. Nemiah JC: Dissociative disorders, in Comprehensive Textbook of Psychiatry, 3rd ed. Edited by Freedman AM, Kaplan HI. Baltimore, Williams and Wilkins, 1981

8. American Psychiatric Association: Diagnostic and Statistical Manual of Mental Disorders (Third Edition). Washington, DC, American Psychiatric Association, 1980

9. Abeles M, Schilder P: Psychogenic loss of personal identity. Archives of Neurology and Psychiatry 34:587-604, 1935

10. Kanzer M: Amnesia: a statistical study. Am J Psychiatry 96:711-716, 1939

11. Kennedy A, Neville J: Sudden loss of memory. Br Med J 2:428-433, 1957

12. Kiersch TA: Amnesia: a clinical study of ninety-eight cases. Am J Psychiatry 119:57-60, 1962

13. Rosen H, Myers H: Abreaction in the military setting. Archives of Neurology and Psychiatry 57:161-172, 1947

14. Berrington WP, Liddell DW, Foulds GA: A re-evaluation of the fugue. Journal of Mental Sciences 102:280-286, 1956

15. Slater E, Roth M: Clinical Psychiatry, 3rd ed. Baltimore, Williams and Wilkins, 1974

16. Akhtar S, Brenner I: Differential diagnosis of fugue-like states. J Clin Psychiatry 40:381-385, 1979

17. Mayeux R, Alexander MP, Benson F, et al: Poriomania. Neurology 29:1616-1619, 1979

18. Fisher C: The psychogenesis of fugue states. Am J Psychother 1:211-220, 1947

19. Luparello TJ: Features of fugue: a unified hypothesis of regression. J Am Psychoanal Assoc 18:379-398, 1970

20. Janet P: The Major Symptoms of Hysteria. New York, Macmillan, 1890

21. Dixon JC: Depersonalization phenomena in a sample population of college students. Br J Psychiatry 109:371-375, 1963

22. Freud S: A disturbance of memory on the acropolis. Int J Psychoanal 22:93-101, 1941

23. Stamm JL: The problems of depersonalization in Freud's "Disturbance of memory on the acropolis." American Imago 26:364-372, 1969

24. Cattell JP: Depersonalization phenomena, in American Handbook of Psychiatry. Edited by Arieti S. New York, Basic Books, 1972

25. Bliss EL: Multiple personalities: a report of 14 cases with implications for schizophrenia and hysteria. Arch Gen Psychiatry 37:1388-1397, 1980

26. Taylor WS, Martin MF: Multiple personality. Journal of Abnormal and Social Psychology 39:281-300, 1944

27. Sutcliffe JP, Jones J: Personal identity, multiple personality, and hypnosis. Int J Clin Exp Hypn 10:231-269, 1962

28. Ludwig AM, Brandsma JM, Wilbur CB, et al: The objective study of a multiple personality, or, are four heads better than one? Arch Gen Psychiatry 26:298-310, 1972

29. Coons PM: Multiple personality: diagnostic consideration. J Clin Psychiatry 41:330-336, 1980

30. Boor M, Coons PM: A comprehensive bibliography of literature pertaining to multiple personality. Psychol Rep 53:295-310, 1983

31. Ellenberger HF: The Discovery of the Unconscious: The History and Evolution of Dynamic Psychiatry. New York, Basic Books, 1970

32. Rosenbaum M: The role of the term schizophrenia in the decline of diagnoses of multiple personality. Arch Gen Psychiatry 37:1383-1385, 1980

33. Braun BG: Foreword to symposium on multiple personality. Psychiatr Clin North Am 7:1-2, 1984

34. Kluft RP: Treatment of multiple personality disorder: a study of 33 cases. Psychiatr Clin North Am 7:9-29, 1984

35. Horevitz RP, Braun BG: Are multiple personalities borderline? Psychiatr Clin North Am 7:69-88, 1984

36. Putnam FW, Post RM, Guroff JJ, et al: 100 cases of multiple personality disorder. Presented at American Psychiatric Association Annual Meeting, New Research Abstract #77. New York, April 30-May 6, 1983

37. Henderson JL, Moore M: The psychoneuroses of war. New Engl J Med 230:273-279, 1944

38. Archibald HC, Tuddenham RD: Persistent stress reaction after combat: a 20 year follow-up. Arch Gen Psychiatry 12:475-481, 1965

39. Ewalt JR, Crawford D: Posttraumatic stress syndrome. Curr Psychiatr Ther 20:145-153, 1981

40. Sargent W, Slater E: Amnesic syndromes in war. Proceedings of the Royal Society of Medicine 34:757-764, 1941

41. Torrie A: Psychosomatic casualties in the Middle East. Lancet 29:139-143, 1944

42. Grinker RR, Spiegel JP: War Neuroses in North Africa. New York, Josiah Macy Jr Foundation, 1943

43. Fisher C: Amnesic states in war neuroses: the psychogenesis of fugues. Psychoanal Q 14:437-468, 1945

44. Kirshner LA: Dissociative reactions: an historical review and clinical study. Acta Psychiatr Scand 49:698-711, 1973

45. Herold CM: Critical analysis of the elements of psychic functions: Part I. Psychoanal Q 10:513-544, 1941

46. Geleerd ER, Hacker FJ, Rapaport D: Contribution to the study of amnesia and allied conditions. Psychoanal Q 14:199-220, 1945

47. Geleerd ER: Clinical contribution to the problem of the early mother-child relationship. Psychoanal Study Child 11:336-351, 1956

48. Stengel E: Further studies on pathological wandering (fugues with the impulse to wander). Journal of the Mental Sciences 89:224-241, 1943

49. Stengel E: On the aetiology of fugue states. Journal of the Mental Sciences 87:572-599, 1941

50. Stengel E: Studies on the psychopathology of compulsive wandering: a preliminary report. Br J Med Psychol 18:250-254, 1939

51. Wilson G, Rupp C: Amnesia. Am J Psychiatry 106:481-485, 1950

52. Acker B: Depersonalization: I. Aetiology and phenomenology; II. Clinical syndromes. Journal of the Mental Sciences 100:836-872, 1954

53. Lewis A: Melancholia: a clinical survey of depressive states. Journal of the Mental Sciences 80:277-278, 1934

54. Roth M: The phobic-anxiety-depersonalization syndrome. Proceedings of the Royal Society of Medicine 52:587-595, 1959

55. Torch EM: Review of the relationship between obsession and depersonalization. Acta Psychiatr Scand 58:191-198, 1978

56. Szymanski HV: Prolonged depersonalization after marijuana use. Am J Psychiatry 138:231-233, 1981

57. Bliss EL, Clark LD, West CD: Studies in sleep-deprivation—relationship to schizophrenia. Archives of Neurology and Psychiatry 81:348-359, 1959

58. Penfield W, Kriestiensen K: Epileptic Seizure Patterns. Springfield, Il, Charles C Thomas, 1951

59. Simpson J: The clinical neurology of temporal lobe disorders, in Current Problems in Neuropsychiatry. Edited by Herrington R. London, Br J Psychiatry, Special Publications No. 4, 1969

60. Roberts W: Normal and abnormal depersonalization. Journal of the Mental Sciences 106:478-493, 1960

61. Sedman G: Depersonalization in a group of normal subjects. Br J Psychiatry 112:907-912, 1966

62. Harper M: Deja vu and depersonalization in normal subjects. Aust NZ J Psychiatry 3:67-74, 1969

63. Myers D, Grant G: A study of depersonalization in students. Br J Psychiatry 121:59-65, 1970

64. Jacobson E: Depersonalization. J Am Psychoanal Assoc 7:581-609, 1977

65. Bettelheim B: The individual and mass behavior in extreme situations, in Surviving and Other Essays. New York, Harcourt, 1979

66. Krystal H: Massive Psychic Trauma. New York, International Universities Press, 1969

67. Bluhm H: How did they survive? Am J Psychother 2:3-32, 1949

68. Dor-Shav KN: On the long-range effects of concentration camp internment on Nazi victims: 35 years later. J Consult Clin Psychol 46:1-11, 1978

69. Noyes R, Kletti R: Depersonalization in response to life-threatening danger. Psychiatry 18:375-384, 1977

70. Noyes R, Hoenk PR, Kupperman BA, et al: Depersonalization in accident victims and psychiatric patients. J Nerv Ment Dis 164:401-407, 1977

71. Noyes R, Slymen DJ: The subjective response to life-threatening danger. Omega 9:313-321, 1978-1979

72. Breuer J, Freud S: Studies in Hysteria. New York, Basic Books, 1957

73. Fliess R: The hypnotic evasion: a clinical observation. Psychoanal Q 22: 497-511, 1953

74. Loewald HW: Hypnoid state, repression, abreaction and recollection. J Am Psychoanal Assoc 3:201-210, 1955

75. Dickes R: The defensive function of an altered state of consciousness: a hypnoid state. J Am Psychoanal Assoc 13:356-403, 1965

76. Silber A: Childhood seduction, parental pathology and hysterical symptomatology: the genesis of an altered state of consciousness. Int J Psychoanal 60:109-116, 1979

77. Fagan J, McMahon PP: Incipient multiple personality in children: four cases. J Nerv Ment Dis 172:6-36, 1984

78. Kluft RP: Multiple personality in childhood. Psychiatr Clin North Am 7:3-8, 1984

79. Wilbur CB: Multiple personality and child abuse. Psychiatr Clin North Am 7:3-8, 1984

80. Saltman V, Solomon RS: Incest and multiple personality. Psychol Rep 50:1127-1141, 1982

81. Stern CR: The etiology of multiple personalities. Psychiatr Clin North Am 7:149-160, 1984

82. Kluft RP: Personal communication, October 1984

83. Mayer-Gross W: On depersonalization. Br J Med Psychol 15:103-126, 1936

84. Shorvon HJ: The depersonalization syndrome. Proceedings of the Royal Society of Medicine 39:779-792, 1946

85. Davison K: Episodic depersonalization: observations on 7 patients. Br J Psychiatry 110:505-513, 1984

86. Brauer R, Harrow M, Tucker GJ: Depersonalization phenomena in psychiatric patients. Br J Psychiatry 117:509-515, 1970

87. Tucker GJ, Harrow M, Zuinlan D: Depersonalization, dysphoria and thought disturbance. Am J Psychiatry 130:702-706, 1973

88. Fleiss JL, Gurland BJ, Goldberg K: Independence of depersonalization-derealization. J Consult Clin Psychol 43:110-111, 1975

89. Parikh MD, Sheth AS, Apte JS: Depersonalization: a phenomenological study in psychiatric patients. J Postgrad Med 27:226-230, 1981

90. Allison RB: A new treatment approach for multiple personalities. Am J Clin Hypn 17:15-32, 1974

91. Gittleson NL: A phenomenological test of a theory of depersonalization. Br J Psychiatry 113:677-678, 1967

92. Nuller YL: Depersonalization—symptoms, meaning, therapy. Acta Psychiatr Scand 66:451-458, 1982

93. Kluft RP: An introduction to multiple personality disorder. Psychiatric Annals 14:19-26, 1984

94. Bliss EL: Spontaneous self-hypnosis in multiple personality disorder. Psychiatr Clin North Am 7:135-148, 1984

95. Putnam FW, Loewenstein RJ, Silberman EK, et al: Multiple personality disorder in a hospital setting. J Clin Psychiatry 45:172-175, 1984

96. Hwu HG, Chen CC, Tsuang MT, et al: Derealization syndrome and the outcome of schizophrenia: a report from the international pilot study of schizophrenia. Br J Psychiatry 139:313-318, 1981

97. Oberndorf CP: The role of anxiety in depersonalization. Int J Psychoanal 31:1-5, 1950

98. Torch EM: Depersonalization syndrome: an overview. Psychiatr Q 53:249-258, 1981

99. Jackson H: On seizures. Brain 22:534-549, 1899

100. Penfield W, Jasper H: Epilepsy and the Functional Anatomy of the Human Brain. Boston, Little Brown and Co., 1954

101. Fullerton DT, Harvy RF, Klein MH, et al: Psychiatric disorders in patients with spinal cord injuries. Arch Gen Psychiatry 38:1369-1371, 1981

102. Clary WF, Burstin KJ, Carpenter JS: Multiple personality and borderline personality disorder. Psychiatr Clin North Am 7:89-100, 1984

103. Salfield DJ: Depersonalization and allied disturbances in childhood. Journal of the Mental Sciences 104:472-476, 1958

104. Fast I, Chethik M: Aspects of depersonalization-derealization in the experience of children. International Review of Psychoanalysis 3:438-490, 1976

105. Hilgard ER: Divided Consciousness: Multiple Controls in Human Thought and Action. New York, John Wiley and Sons, 1977

106. Ambrose G: Hypnotherapy with Children. London, Staples Press, 1961

107. London P: Developmental experiments in hypnosis. Journal of Prospective Techniques and Personality Assessment 29:189-199, 1965

108. London P, Cooper LM: Norms of hypnotic susceptibility in children. Developmental Psychology 1:113-124, 1969

109. Gardiner GG: Hypnosis with children and adolescents. Int J Clin Exp Hypn 22:20-38, 1974

110. Williams DT: Hypnosis as a psychotherapeutic adjunct with children and adolescents. Psychiatric Annals 11:47-54, 1981

111. Place M: Hypnosis and the child. J Child Psychol Psychiatry 25:339-347, 1984

112. Gardiner GG: Hypnosis with infants and preschool children. Am J Clin Hypn 19:158-162, 1977

113. Nowlis DP: The child-rearing antecedents of hypnotic susceptibility and of naturally occurring hypnotic-like experience. Int J Clin Exp Hypn 17:109-120, 1969

114. Hilgard ER: Personality and Hypnosis: A Study of Imaginative Involvement. Chicago, University of Chicago Press, 1970

115. Cooper LM, London P: Children's hypnotic susceptibility, personality and EEG patterns. Int J Clin Hypn 24:140-148, 1976

116. Svendsen M: Children's imaginary companions. Archives of Neurology and Psychiatry 32:985-999, 1934

117. Pines M: Invisible playmates. Psychology Today 106:38-42, 1976

118. Baum EA: Imaginary companions of two children. J Am Acad Child Psychiatry 32:324-330, 1978

119. Myers WA: Imaginary companions, fantasy twins, mirror dreams and depersonalization. J Am Psychoanal Assoc 45:503-524, 1976

5

The Relationship Among Dissociation, Hypnosis, and Child Abuse in the Development of Multiple Personality Disorder

Edward J. Frischholz, M.A.

5

The Relationship Among Dissociation, Hypnosis, and Child Abuse in the Development of Multiple Personality Disorder

The study of the relationships among dissociation, hypnosis, and multiple personality disorder can be traced to the work of Janet (1) and Prince (2) at the end of the 19th and the beginning of the 20th century. Both hypnosis and multiple personality disorder are considered to be forms of dissociative phenomena (3–5). The current Diagnostic and Statistical Manual of Mental Disorders, Third Edition (DSM-III) (6) includes multiple personality disorder among the dissociative disorders. For almost a century, hypnosis has been explained as a form of dissociation (1, 2, 4, 7). For decades, clinicians have implicitly linked dissociation, hypnosis, and multiple personality disorder by assuming that multiple personality disorder patients are more hypnotizable than other clinical groups (2, 5, 8).

More recently, clinicians (9, 10) and researchers (11, 12) have identified an association between the severity of the childhood punishment an individual has endured, and that individual's hypnotic responsivity. This relates to efforts to understand the defensive functions of dissociation and its use as a coping and/or defense mechanism in multiple personality disorder (3, 5, 13, 14). These lines of thinking hypothesize that a traumatic event (such

The author would like to thank Dr. Richard P. Kluft for his assistance in the preparation of this chapter.

as child abuse) may stimulate a state of overwhelming anxiety, to which the individual with dissociative capacity may respond defensively by dissociating aspects or the entirety of his or her conscious experience of the traumatic event. Some workers surmise that the conjunction of hypnotizability (15) or dissociation-proneness (14) with child abuse or other overwhelming circumstances is related to the development of multiple personality disorder.

This chapter will evaluate theories and empirical evidence that have been offered to clarify (as well as to refute) the relations among dissociation, hypnosis, and multiple personality disorder. I will begin by examining the concept of dissociation and its relation to multiple personality disorder. Next, I will assess the evidence that relates hypnosis to the concept of dissociation, focusing on the differential hypnotizability of multiple personality disorder patients in comparison to other clinical groups. Then, I will consider the role of early traumatic events, particularly child abuse, in relation to hypnotic responsivity and the development of multiple personality disorder. In conclusion, I will attempt to summarize and integrate these theories and experimental findings and indicate directions for potential future research.

THE CONCEPT OF DISSOCIATION AND MULTIPLE PERSONALITY DISORDER

To dissociate means to sever the association of one thing from another. Janet (1) formulated this conceptualization in order to describe and explain certain phenomena he observed among his patients. Dissociation was derived from the doctrine of association, which was the most widely accepted theory of human memory during Janet's era. This theory proposed that memories were brought to consciousness through the association of ideas. Things which could not be remembered were said to be "dissociated."

Why was the concept of dissociation necessary? Janet observed that some of his patients appeared to have dual or multiple personalities. Each different personality had a life history of his or her own. Information learned by one personality was not always consciously available to the other personality or personalities. He saw that a particular patient might behave differently on various occasions, and found that this variance in behavior appeared to correlate with the emergences of the various personalities. Thus, each personality seemed to have its own set of memories and its characteristic behavioral style. A distinctive feature of this syndrome was the amnesia of one personality for information learned by another personality. Janet regarded the inaccessible memories as "dissociated" from and unavailable to the conscious experience of the patient at a given point in time. Thus, the concept of "dissociation" was originally necessary to explain and describe some of the phenomena of multiple personality disorder.

The above observations led Janet to speculate that consciousness flowed in many streams, which did not necessarily flow together. Information that entered consciousness via one stream could not always be assumed to be available or accessible to other streams. The concept of dissociation seemed to explain how the different personalities could coexist within the same physical body without awareness of one another.

The theory that information can be processed without conscious awareness was advanced by a number of workers prior to the 20th century (15). Both Janet and Freud had postulated that such "unconscious" processing could affect ongoing conscious behavior without the subject's awareness of the source of this influence. However, when Freud extended Cartesian dualism into the topographical construct of conscious/unconscious, he identified repression instead of dissociation as the mechanism by which information was rendered inaccessible to conscious experience. Since repression seemed to explain the behavior of both multiple personality disorder and nonmultiple personality disorder patients, it was considered to be the more universal construct. Dissociation became regarded as a specific form of repression (7). A number of contemporary authors have studied the history of the relationship between dissociation and repression (4, 7, 16).

Following Janet's and Freud's formulations, the existence of the unconscious appeared to gain widespread popular acceptance. However, it was not welcomed uncritically among the academic medical community. Ellenberger offers a fascinating description of how these ideas were received by the medical establishment of the time (15). While some reasons for misgivings had to do with controversies surrounding other issues these investigators (especially Freud) had raised, the prevailing medical *zeitgeist* held that a truly scientific account of human consciousness should be firmly grounded in physiology. Since both repression and dissociation were psychological explanations, neither fulfilled the above criterion. Hence, both concepts were regarded as unscientific.

Morton Prince was the next major investigator to study dissociation. His analysis of Miss Beauchamp was summarized in *The Dissociation of a Personality* (2). Both there and in his later experimental studies with multiple personality disorder patients (17), some of which involved hypnosis, Prince concluded that it was "inconceivable" that a purely physiological explanation could account for the symptoms observed in multiple personality disorder.

Despite Prince's studies, both the concept of dissociation and the diagnosis of multiple personality disorder fell into disrepute. Rosenbaum (18) surmises that the two primary reasons for this decline in interest were: 1) Bleuler's introduction of the term "schizophrenia," under the rubric of which were many symptoms shared by this disorder and multiple personality disorder; and 2) multiple personality disorder, like hysteria, came to be regarded as an artifact of hypnotic suggestion, and hence was not perceived to be a genuine diagnostic entity. Bleuler's formulation of schizophrenia was more in keeping with the medical *zeitgeist* of this period. It assumed that there was an underlying deterioration in physiological functioning which caused and became manifest in the deficits in adaptive behavior shown by schizophrenic individuals. Rosenbaum has argued that the decline in the number of cases diagnosed as multiple personality disorder between 1910 and 1970 may be due to the fact that many multiple personality disorder patients were incorrectly diagnosed as schizophrenic (18).

Recently, the contention that multiple personality disorder is an artifact of hypnotic suggestion has been questioned on two grounds (19, 20). First, multiple personality disorder has been observed in a large number of patients who had no previous exposure to hypnosis. Second, hypnotically created entities described as "multiple personalities" are qualitatively different from the additional personalities observed in multiple personality disorder patients. These induced entities have no previous life history and serve no particular adaptive function. A related concern is that a series of psychological experiments conducted between 1925 and 1945 suggested that hypnosis could not be characterized adequately as a form of dissociation (by implication) similar to that which was observed in multiple personality disorder (21–23). These reports and more recent studies bearing on this topic will be discussed in the next section.

The decline of reported multiple personality disorder cases from 1910 to 1970 was probably also influenced by changes in the newly expanding field of psychology. During the 1920s through the 1950s, psychology was heavily influenced by the behaviorist views of Watson, Hull, and Skinner. As a result, many psychologists preferred to focus on fluctuations in observed behavior rather than reported alterations in conscious experience. This turning away from the study of experience may have contributed to facilitating psychologists' misdiagnosis of multiple personality disorder.

Taylor and Martin's 1944 article reviewed 76 documented cases of multiple personality disorder (24). That such a small number of cases could be retrieved from the world's literature strengthened the general belief that the incidence of this disorder was extremely rare. The first two editions of the Diagnostic and Statistical Manual of Mental Disorders (25, 26) categorized multiple personality disorder as a variety of hysterical neurosis, choosing not to accord it a separate classification. Although the movie [the] *Three Faces of Eve*, based on an actual case study (27), brought a brief spurt of popular and professional attention to the syndrome, neither it nor the articles written about "Eve" succeeded in generating scientific interest in multiple personality disorder.

Multiple personality disorder received little attention in the scientific literature from 1960 through 1975. However, beginning in the 1960s, there was a rebirth of interest in the concept of dissociation (4, 7, 28). This renewed attention paralleled a rise in the influence of the humanistic school of psychology, which accepted a person's description of his or her conscious experiences as valid scientific data. Several different types of dissociation have now been studied. In general, they can be classified into two broad categories: 1) dissociations of consciousness or awareness; and 2) dissociations of volitional control. Unfortunately, almost all of the recent empirical research on these forms of dissociation has been conducted in the environment of the hypnosis laboratory. Only recently have attempts been made to study clinical multiple personality disorder as a naturally occurring form of dissociation.

One major reason why the laboratory investigation of hypnosis became the preferred method of studying dissociation is that highly hypnotizable subjects have been more readily available than multiple personality disorder patients. Until the late 1970s the incidence of multiple personality disorder was considered to be quite rare. Ralph B. Allison, M.D. (29) was one of the first mental health professionals to point out the difficulties associated with making the diagnosis of multiple personality disorder. He surmised that this syndrome might be more common than was previously suspected.

DSM-III facilitated the study of multiple personality disorder by identifying it as a dissociative disorder distinct from the hysterical neuroses, and establishing diagnostic criteria (6). However, it continued to describe the prevalence of multiple personality disorder as "extremely rare." To my knowledge, no attempt has yet been undertaken to use the DSM-III criteria in a study to estimate the incidence and prevalence of multiple personality disorder.

There is evidence accumulating, however, which indicates that multiple personality disorder may be more common than earlier estimates had suggested. At the First International Conference on Multiple Personality/Dissociative States held in Chicago in September 1984, the scientific program's 92 contributors collectively had seen over 400 separate documented cases of multiple personality disorder in the last decade. Seventy professionals at a course there had seen an additional 267 (see Kluft's Introduction to this monograph). These figures stand in sharp contrast to the 76 documented cases in the world literature reported 30 years before by Taylor and Martin (24).

In the last five years, several clinicians have begun to study series of multiple personality disorder cases, declining to engage in building elaborate theories from single case studies (14, 20, 30, 31).

These reports have focused primarily on such issues as the demographic characteristics of multiple personality disorder patients and their response to treatment. Braun's chapter on the transgenerational incidence of multiple personality disorder (Chapter 6 of this monograph) is one of the first attempts to identify commonalities among the family histories of multiple personality disorder patients. His findings suggest that there are both genetic and environmental determinants of this disorder. This type of process-oriented analysis will further clarify our understanding of the concept of dissociation and its role in the development of multiple personality disorder.

What have we learned about dissociation since Janet's time? As stated earlier, most empirical studies on dissociation have been conducted in the context of laboratory experiments in hypnosis. The systematic study of dissociation in multiple personality disorder patients is only beginning. There are, however, some definitive statements that can be made about dissociation as a heuristic construct.

The original concept of dissociation was based on the notion that information being processed at one level of awareness (conscious/unconscious) should not interfere with information being processed at another level of awareness. Early experiments performed by both Janet (1) and Prince (17) seemed to support this notion of noninterference. The most frequent experimental design consisted of hypnotizing the subjects and suggesting that posthypnotic automatic writing was to be carried out following a prearranged signal. Subjects were also instructed that they would have no memory for this suggestion and would not be aware that they were writing. Hypnosis was then terminated. The prearranged cue was administered after a short delay. Using this design with his patient, Lucie, Janet observed that her hand began to write following the signal, although she was carrying on a casual conversation at the time.

Later, when Janet showed her the letter she had written, she was unable to comprehend how it had been produced. She believed that Janet had copied her handwriting. The fact that Lucie could unconsciously engage in writing a legible and comprehensible letter while conversing about another topic was interpreted to mean that the automatic writing did not interfere with her ongoing conscious behavior. Unfortunately, the criterion of noninterference gradually became the empirical test for the validity of dissociation as a psychological construct.

A series of studies carried out from 1925 to 1945 clearly indicated that subjects who were hypnotically instructed to be amnesic for certain information still showed evidence of profiting from this information when tested while no longer hypnotized (21–23). These investigators concluded that hypnotic amnesia did not produce a functional interference between the unconscious processing of information and ongoing behavior. Hence, hypnosis was not considered to be adequately characterized as a form of dissociation.

Close examination of the criterion of noninterference, however, indicates that it is not an appropriate method for testing the presence of dissociation. As noted earlier, the concept of dissociation was originally formulated in order to understand the cognitions and behaviors of multiple personality disorder patients. The various personalities usually have some awareness for some information learned by other personalities. This clearly violates the criterion of non-interference. Yet, it is an observable phenomenon in the very type of patient that stimulated the formulation of the concept of dissociation.

At present, it now seems much more informative to document the degree of functional amnesia which exists among the various personalities in any multiple personality disorder patient, rather than to consider all memories as functionally inaccessible. Similarly, it would be informative to know how well the degree of noninterference correlates with measured hypnotizability. If hypnosis is to be appropriately characterized as a form of dissociation, the more hypnotizable subjects should show a higher level of noninterference between tasks performed at different levels of awareness. We will discuss this issue in detail in the next section.

What major questions remain to be answered about the explanatory power of dissociation as a psychological construct? First, if dissociation is presumed to be a psychological defense mechanism, then it should be clearly differentiated from other defense mechanisms, particularly the Freudian concept of repression. Hilgard (4) has proposed that the major difference between the two concepts concerns the flow and content of the dissociated/repressed material. In a dissociation conceptualization, there is an amnesic barrier that prevents the interchange of different memories. However, in a repression formulation, there is only an amnesia for unacceptable impulses.

Spiegel (7) has emphasized the two-directional nature of dissociation and prefers to speak of a "dissociation-association continuum." Repression, in contrast, is regarded as a one-directional concept. For example, the associations available to everyday awareness are necessary for sustaining attention in order to make adaptive responses. Repression occurs when conscious awareness of an internal or external object is psychologically constricted. However, awareness can also be expanded so that what is dissociated becomes associated or integrated into a more mature psychological system. Ultimately, the use of dissociation as a psychological defense will have to be studied systematically in multiple personality disorder patients in order to more fully understand how information becomes selectively associated or dissociated from conscious experience.

In summary, to dissociate means to sever the association of one thing from another. This conceptualization was originally formulated by Janet in order to explain the symptoms of multiple personality disorder (1). Interest in both dissociation and multiple personality disorder has waxed and waned over the last 100 years, during which hypnosis has been the most extensively studied form of dissociation. More recent reports have suggested that the incidence of multiple personality disorder may be much higher than was previously suspected. Already, some clinicians/investigators are beginning to study consecutive series of multiple personality disorder cases, instead of theorizing elaborately on the basis of single case studies. It is hoped that this will stimulate a more process-oriented analysis of dissociation as it occurs naturally. The criterion of noninterference of information processing, which occurs at different levels of awareness, was shown to be an inadequate test of the presence of dissociation, because some interference of information can usually be observed in multiple personality disorder patients. Finally, we need to know more about how dissociation operates as a psychological defense mechanism in protecting the psychological system from overwhelming anxiety. In the next section, I will identify what we have learned about dissociation and multiple personality disorder through experiments involving hypnosis.

HYPNOSIS AS A FORM OF DISSOCIATION

What is hypnosis? Although there is no universally agreed upon definition of this phenomenon, there is some consensus that the hypnotized subject reports alterations in perception and/or memory that momentarily become credible (28, 32, 33). This description focuses on a major point of agreement among contemporary researchers and clinicians regarding what is characteristic of hypnosis. Current scientific theories about hypnosis have differed in their explanations about how these alterations in perception and/or memory take place. For example, hypnosis has been described as a "goal-directed imagining" by Spanos and Barber (34), as "role enactment" by Sarbin and Coe (35), as a form of "focused concentration" by Spiegel and Spiegel (5), and in terms of "neodissociation theory" by Hilgard (4). However, all these theories acknowledge that credible fluctuations in perception and/or memory take place among hypnotizable subjects.

Why is hypnosis considered a form of dissociation? The major reason is that hypnosis, like dissociation, has been historically associated with changes in awareness, memory, and volition. Experiments that utilized the noninterference criterion claimed that hypnosis was inappropriately characterized as a form of dissociation. However, some investigators have realized that the noninterference criterion itself was inappropriate, and a neodissociation interpretation of hypnotic behavior has recently been offered by Hilgard (4).

What have we learned about dissociation from the experiments on hypnosis? These experiments have addressed several important questions, including: 1) Is hypnosis/dissociation a universal human phenomenon? 2) What accounts for individual differences in hypnotizability and dissociative ability? 3) What have experiments on hypnosis taught us about dissociations in human awareness and volitional control? 4) Lastly, how hypnotizable are multiple personality disorder patients in reference to other clinical groups? Each of these questions will be considered separately in the sections below.

Is Hypnosis/Dissociation a Universal Human Phenomenon?

Clinical observation and research carried out over the last century has clearly documented that there are wide individual differences in the ability to become hypnotized (5, 28). Additional research has documented that these individual differences in hypnotizability are stable over time (36, 37). Those experiments that have attempted to modify subjects' responsivity to hypnosis have been largely unsuccessful. Any changes observed have been small, although some achieved statistical significance (38). However, it has also been observed that subjects in such modification experiments maintain their same relative standing in the overall distribution of hypnotizability (39, 40). This means that while there is some variation in absolute hypnotic responsivity across different measurement contexts, for most purposes subjects found to be unresponsive in one context will earn lower hypnotizability scores in other contexts, as well. Collectively, these studies indicate that hypnotic responsivity or hypnotizability is best characterized as an ability that people possess in varying degrees. This leads us to infer that there are also wide individual differences in the ability to dissociate.

The observation that there are wide individual differences in hypnotizability seems at variance with the claims of many clinical practitioners that everyone is hypnotizable (41, 42). This claim, however, can be shown to be based on the assumption that hypnosis necessarily follows an hypnotic induction ceremony. Therefore, if an hypnotic induction ceremony was administered, then the patient surely must have been hypnotized. However, as noted above, there are wide individual differences in the capacity to enter a trance. Some people are incapable of responding to a hypnotic induction ceremony. Further close examination of the claim that everyone is hypnotizable reveals that most clinicians who hold this belief think that all patients are capable of responding to "hypnotic treatment" or "hypnotherapy." Elsewhere, this author has argued that hypnosis should not be considered as a form of treatment or therapy in its own right (43; see also, discussions in 44–47). Rather, hypnosis should be considered ancillary to a primary treatment strategy such as psychoanalysis, systematic desensitization, or cognitive restructuring.

It seems as if those clinicians who maintain that everyone is hypnotizable might be understood as saying that most people are capable of profiting from some form of treatment. This is tantamount to equating hypnotic responsivity with treatment responsivity. However, these two concepts are different, and not interchangeable. It seems far more revealing to see if individual differences in hypnotic responsivity are predictive of individual differences in treatment outcome. Indeed, some studies have already appeared that support this contention (48, 49).

What Accounts for Individual Differences in Hypnotizability?

There is neither consensus nor certainty regarding all the variables that contribute to individual differences in hypnotizability. Morgan (50) conducted a twin study in the hopes of identifying a genetic factor. Her findings indicated that there were higher correlations between the hypnotizability scores of monozygotic twins than between dizygotic twins or other family members. These results are consistent with a genetic interpretation, and suggest that individual differences in the ability to dissociate may be determined, in part, by subjects' heredity. However, the correlations were not high enough to consider heredity as the sole determinant of individual differences in hypnotic performance.

Another finding that emerges from work over the last 20 years is that imaginative involvement or absorption is significantly associated with hypnotic responsivity (11, 51). Imaginative involvement/absorption is a personality trait that refers to a subject's ability to become so involved/absorbed in a particular activity that his or her peripheral awareness becomes significantly diminished. For example, subjects may become so involved in watching a movie that they lose awareness of what is going on around them. When the movie is over, subjects who score high on measures of imaginative involvement/absorption may have become so involved/absorbed that they may be somewhat surprised to find that they are in a movie theater. The cause of individual differences in imaginative involvement/absorption is unknown.

Josephine Hilgard (11), in an extensive interview study, found that a sum of imaginative involvement ratings correlated r (185) = .35, $p < .001$ with scores on the Stanford Hypnotic Susceptibility Scale, Form C (SHSS:C) (52). As with the findings from Morgan's twin study (50), this correlation is not high enough to consider imaginative involvement/absorption as the only correlate of individual differences in hypnotizability. In fact, future research may find that individual differences in both hypnotizability and imaginative involvement/absorption are determined by similar genetic and environmental factors.

An unexpected finding to emerge from J. Hilgard's interview study (11) was that the subject's rating of the severity of the punishment he or she had received as a child was correlated r (185) = .30, $p < .001$ with SHSS:C scores. However, the association between the punishment rating and the sum of the imaginative involvement ratings was a statistically insignificant correlation of .12. This indicates that imaginative involvement and severity of punishment ratings are relatively independent predictors of measured hypnotic responsivity. In order to test this hypothesis, I performed two additional analyses of J. Hilgard's data. First, the technique of partial correlation was used to determine the association between the severity of punishment ratings and the SHSS:C scores after controlling for the confounding variance of imaginative involvement ratings. This partial correlation was found to be .28 ($p < .01$), which is very similar to the simple correlation of .30 observed between SHSS:C scores and imaginative involvement.

In the second analysis, a multiple correlation was calculated using a linear combination of imaginative involvement ratings and severity of punishment ratings to predict SHSS:C scores. The F statistic was then used to determine whether the two predictor variables yielded a significantly better prediction of SHSS:C scores than emerged from using imaginative involvement ratings alone as the predictor. The multiple correlation was .44 and the F statistic (F (1,184) = 14.2, $p < .001$) indicated that utilizing both predictor variables resulted in a significant increase in the prediction of SHSS:C scores relative to using a single predictor variable. This summary is not intended to identify all of the variables that have been found to be predictive of hypnotizability. Instead, as the statistical analyses performed above clearly indicate, individual differences in hypnotizability are most likely to be determined by multiple factors. Similarly, individual differences in dissociative ability are probably determined by many factors. Future research will be needed to identify the most salient determinants of hypnotizability and the ability to dissociate.

Hypnosis and Dissociations in Awareness and Volitional Control

Historically, hypnosis has been associated with dissociations in awareness and volitional control. In fact, these variables have been used to determine whether a subject was indeed hypnotized. Many items on current measures of hypnotic responsivity are directly related to these phenomena. Hull (21) and Hilgard (4, 28) have thoroughly reviewed most of the experimental studies in this area. The interested reader is referred to these sources for a more detailed discussion of this topic. In the present section, we will only consider the perceived involuntariness of motor behavior during hypnosis and recent studies on the phenomenon of the "hidden observer" (4).

Dissociations of Volitional Control and Hypnosis

Most measures of hypnotic responsivity include items that assess the subject's motor response to an hypnotic suggestion.

Usually, such items are scored on the basis of the subject's behavioral response. The arm lowering item on the widely used SHSS:C (52) is a typical example. The hypnotized subject is instructed to imagine a heavy object in his or her outstretched arm. Instructions are then given that the subject's arm is getting heavier and heavier, and the item is scored as a pass if the subject moves the indicated arm down more than 6 inches below the original starting position. This item is quite easy. Approximately 92 percent of the SHSS:C standardization sample ($N = 203$) passed it. It is assumed that the behavioral response to this suggestion is experienced by the subject as being involuntary.

Recently, Weitzenhoffer, the senior author of all of the Stanford Hypnotic Susceptibility Scales, has claimed that it is unwarranted to assume that a perceived involuntariness accompanies such behavioral responses (53). In data deleted from the final draft of his 1980 paper (53), Weitzenhoffer used the subject's verbal report of complete loss of volitional control over the behavioral movement as the sole criterion for passing the item. With this revision, he found that only five percent of his subjects passed the item, which 92 percent of a standardization sample had passed by purely behavioral criteria (52). He concluded that future revisions of the Stanford scales should measure the loss of volitional control more directly (53).

Bowers (54) recently conducted a study bearing directly on the issue of loss of volitional control during hypnotic motor behavior. Twenty-four subjects were administered the Stanford Form A scale (55), which predominantly assesses changes in motor behavior observed during hypnosis. Afterward, each subject was asked to rate his or her perceived involuntariness of response on each item. All subjects were administered the SHSS:C subsequently. Results indicated that the SHSS:A behavioral score correlated .77 with subjects' later SHSS:C scores, and .78 with the sum of the subjects' involuntariness ratings. Bowers (54) concluded that Weitzenhoffer's concerns were unfounded, and that the behavioral response was as good an index of perceived involuntariness as more direct measures of the subjects' volitional control.

A reanalysis of the data in the Bowers report (54) indicates that his conclusion may be unfounded. First, Bowers made little of the fact that the sum of the involuntariness ratings correlated highest ($r = .85$) with SHSS:C scores. Second, analysis of the data using the technique of partial correlation yields a somewhat different picture. The partial correlation between the involuntariness ratings and SHSS:C scores, when one statistically removes the shared variance of the SHSS:A behavioral scores, was highly significant ($r = .63$). This indicates that when the variations in behavioral response are partialed out of the analysis, there remains a highly significant association between involuntariness and subsequent SHSS:C scores. Thus, Weitzenhoffer's concerns (53) are justified, and future research on how hypnosis relates to dissociations in volitional control should utilize more direct measurements of the subjects' perceived volitional experience.

Dissociations in Awareness and Hypnosis

Perhaps the most interesting contemporary attempt to relate hypnosis to dissociations in human awareness has been Hilgard's (4) use of the "hidden observer" metaphor. In a typical hidden observer experiment, subjects are exposed to a noxious stimulus, such as the immersion of one arm in circulating ice water. Baseline pain reports are taken during this period. The subjects are then hypnotized and given hypnotic analgesia instructions. Pain reports are taken during this condition, as well. These pain reports are usually significantly lower than the subjects' baseline pain reports. The hypnotized subjects are then instructed that perhaps there is another part of them, a hidden part, which is still aware of the pain, while the hypnotized part is not. Subjects who report experiencing a hidden observer give pain reports during this condition that are very similar to their baseline pain reports. Hilgard (4) has interpreted this finding as an indication that information can be processed at different levels of awareness. The parallel between this phenomenon and multiple personality disorder is obvious (56).

The major problem with the "hidden observer" phenomenon is that it is very rare. It is found in only approximately 50 percent of very hypnotizable subjects. This means that its incidence in the general population is about five percent. In addition, Spanos and Hewitt (57) have shown that the "hidden observer" can be produced in almost all subjects if these individuals are told to expect its occurrence. However, their study is subject to criticism because it is hardly surprising that the investigators found a phenomenon that they told their subjects they expected to find. A subsequent series of carefully designed studies conducted in Perry's laboratory have confirmed Hilgard's original observations (58, 59). However, more research is necessary before we fully understand the implications of the "hidden observer" phenomenon and its relation to hypnosis and dissociations in awareness.

THE HYPNOTIZABILITY OF MULTIPLE PERSONALITY DISORDER PATIENTS IN RELATION TO OTHER CLINICAL GROUPS

For almost a century, clinicians assumed that multiple personality disorder patients were more hypnotizable than other clinical groups. However, empirical verification of this assumption was lacking. Two independent studies have now addressed this issue. In the first study, Bliss (60) found that the mean SHSS:C score of 28 multiple personality disorder patients (mean = 10.1) was significantly higher than the mean SHSS:C score (mean = 6.6) for a control group of 49 cigarette smokers. This initial study confirmed the hypothesis that multiple personality disorder patients were indeed more hypnotizable than another clinical group.

In a more thorough study of this issue, Frischholz, Lipman, and Braun (61) assessed a sample of multiple personality disorder patients, a sample of heterogeneous clinical patients, and a sample of normal subjects. All subjects were administered both the SHSS:C (52) and Hypnotic Induction Profile (HIP) (5) by two different examiners. Each hypnotizability scale was administered twice, and both examiners were unaware of the diagnosis of the subject when they were testing. Results indicated that hypnotizability scores were reliable and significantly intercorrelated. Multiple personality disorder patients were observed to earn significantly higher mean scores on both measures of hypnotic responsivity than both the clinical and normal samples. In addition, special hypnotic phenomena such as the Hilgard "hidden observer" item were also probed in tests administered to all subjects. The findings indicated that approximately one-half of the multiple personality disorder patients showed the hidden observer phenomenon, while its incidence was extremely rare in the other samples. Kluft found a similar incidence of hidden observer manifestations in an uncontrolled clinical study (62).

The occurrence of the "hidden observer" in multiple personality disorder patients was also found to be closely related to the patients' level of adaptive functioning. Those multiple personality disorder patients who were just beginning treatment all showed a "hidden observer." However, multiple personality disorder patients who had been in treatment for several years showed almost no evidence of this phenomenon. It was almost as if these patients appeared to reject the metaphor of the "hidden observer," perhaps because they were on their way toward integrating their various personalities into a single system.

The studies identified above are among the strongest pieces of evidence that hypnosis is appropriately characterized as one form of dissociation. Patients with a dissociative disorder (that is, multiple personality disorder) were observed to earn higher hypnotizability scores than patients not suffering from a dissociative disorder or normal controls. Why? The most plausible hypothesis is that multiple personality disorder patients find it easier to utilize their capacity to dissociate in a hypnotic setting. Future research is needed to determine whether high hypnotizability is a sufficient condition for developing the symptoms of multiple personality disorder. In the next section, I will argue that it is not.

EARLY TRAUMATIC EVENTS, HYPNOTIZABILITY, AND THE DEVELOPMENT OF MULTIPLE PERSONALITY DISORDER

Kluft (14) indicates that dissociation-proneness, by which he means the biological capacity to dissociate, is one of four factors intrinsic to the etiology of multiple personality disorder. In

Chapter 3 of this monograph, Braun and Sachs offer arguments that a high inborn capacity to dissociate is a necessary but not a sufficient predisposing condition for the development of multiple personality disorder. Their reasoning stems from the observation that not all highly hypnotizable subjects later show symptoms of multiple personality disorder. Instead, they propose that a history of early exposure to various traumatic events is an additional necessary predisposing factor related to the development of this disorder. Both an inborn capacity to dissociate and exposure to overwhelming trauma is necessary, but neither condition by itself is sufficient. One current report offers data that addresses this issue.

Nash et al. (12) recently completed two experiments that were designed to replicate and extend J. Hilgard's (11) earlier observation that subjects' ratings of the severity of their childhood punishments were significantly correlated with adult hypnotic responsivity. In the first study, these experimenters contacted the parents of 14 highly hypnotizable and 11 low hypnotizable subjects regarding the method of discipline used by the parents when the subjects were children. Contrary to previous expectations, low hypnotizable subjects were found to be punished significantly more often than highly hypnotizable subjects.

One reason for the discrepancy between the findings of the J. Hilgard (11) and the Nash et al. (12) study may be that the information regarding childhood punishment came from different sources. In the J. Hilgard study (11), subjects rated the severity of childhood punishment as they remembered it. However, in the Nash et al. study (12), the punishment ratings were made by the subjects' parents instead of by the subjects. This result indicates that it is the subjects' perception of the severity of the punishment they received during childhood that is the important variable. Another viable hypothesis is that parental ratings themselves may be subject to certain pressures toward inaccuracy.

In the second experiment reported by Nash et al. (12), the authors compared the hypnotizability of 16 subjects who were physically abused as children with 300 subjects who were not abused. Results indicated that the abused group earned significantly higher mean hypnotizability scores than the nonabused group. These observations are consistent with J. Hilgard's observations (11).

The findings of J. Hilgard and Nash et al. (12) are consistent with the hypothesis that early childhood abuse is significantly related to adult hypnotic responsivity and, by inference, to dissociative capacity. These results are also congruent with the clinical speculations of Braun and Sachs (15) that early child abuse promotes the use of dissociation as a psychological defense for dealing with traumatic events. The repeated use of dissociation leads to its becoming the individual's primary psychological defense.

It is also obvious that not all children who were abused later develop multiple personality disorder. It is only those children who already have a strong ability to dissociate who make use of this defense mechanism. These are the children who may later become multiple personality disorder patients. The interested reader should turn to Chapter 3 of this monograph for a more detailed discussion of how early childhood trauma, particularly child abuse, combines with the individual's capacity to dissociate, in the development of multiple personality disorder. Kluft has offered a list of traumata other than child abuse that may lead to dissociation (14), and specified nonabuse contributions to defensive dissociation in children in Chapter 8 of this monograph.

SUMMARY

In this chapter, I have attempted to explore the historical relationship between the constructs of dissociation, hypnosis, and multiple personality disorder. The concept of dissociation, which means to sever the association of one thing from another, was originally developed to explain the symptoms of multiple personality disorder. Unfortunately, experiments on the nature of dissociation conducted over the last century have been confined to studies of hypnotic phenomena, because the incidence of multiple personality disorder was considered to be extremely rare.

Evidence collected within the last decade now suggests that

multiple personality disorder may be a much more common syndrome than was previously suspected. The new DSM-III has now identified multiple personality disorder as a "dissociative disorder" distinct from the hysterical neuroses. It is hoped that multiple personality disorder will be more thoroughly studied in the future, and that we will be able to begin to understand the phenomenon of dissociation as it occurs naturally.

Early experiments on hypnosis using the noninterference criterion suggested that hypnosis was not adequately characterized as a form of dissociation. However, more recent thinking has now identified that the noninterference criterion is an inappropriate yardstick. Based on evidence from studies on hypnosis, we can infer that there are wide individual differences in the ability to dissociate, and that these individual differences are determined by many factors. Problems with using hypnosis to study dissociations in volition and awareness were identified, and suggestions for future research were made.

Two recent studies have now confirmed the earlier clinical assumption that multiple personality disorder patients are more hypnotizable than other clinical groups (60, 61). This evidence clearly supports the notion that hypnosis can be appropriately characterized as a form of dissociation.

The relation between child abuse and severity of childhood punishment to later adult hypnotic responsivity has now been documented in two independent laboratories (11, 12). This finding is consistent with the clinical speculations of Braun and Sachs, noted in Chapter 3 of this monograph, that both a strong capacity to dissociate and an early exposure to traumatic events are necessary conditions for the development of multiple personality disorder. Future research should focus on clarifying our understanding of the nature of this relationship.

References

1. Janet P: L'Automatisme Psychologique. Paris, Felix Alcan, 1889

2. Prince M: The Dissociation of a Personality. New York and London, Longmans Green, 1906

3. Braun BG: Towards a theory of multiple personality and other dissociative phenomena. Psychiatr Clin North Am 7:171-194, 1984

4. Hilgard ER: Divided Consciousness: Multiple Controls in Human Thought and Action. New York, John Wiley and Sons, 1977

5. Spiegel H, Spiegel D: Trance and Treatment: Clinical Uses of Hypnosis. New York, Basic Books, 1978

6. American Psychiatric Association: Diagnostic and Statistical Manual of Mental Disorders (Third Edition). Washington, DC, American Psychiatric Association, 1980

7. Spiegel H: The dissociation-association continuum. J Nerv Ment Dis 136:374-378, 1963

8. Winer D: Anger and dissociation: a case study of multiple personality. J Abnorm Psychol 87:368-372, 1978

9. Braun BG: The role of the family in the development of multiple personality disorder. International Journal of Family Psychiatry (in press)

10. Sachs RG, Goodwin J, Braun BG: The role of child abuse in the development of multiple personality disorder, in Multiple Personality and Dissociation. Edited by Braun BG, Kluft RP. New York, Guilford Press (in press)

11. Hilgard J: Personality and hypnosis. Chicago, University of Chicago Press, 1970

12. Nash MR, Lynn SJ, Givens DL: Adult hypnotic susceptibility, childhood punishment, and child abuse: a brief communication. Int J Clin Exp Hypn 32:6-11, 1984

13. Kluft RP: An introduction to multiple personality disorder. Psychiatric Annals 14:21-24, 1984

14. Kluft RP: Treatment of multiple personality. Psychiatr Clin North Am 7:9-29, 1984

15. Ellenberger HF: The Discovery of the Unconscious. New York, Basic Books, 1970

16. Berman E: Multiple personality: psychoanalytic perspective. Int J Psychoanal 62:288-300, 1981

17. Prince M: Experiments to determine co-consciousness (subconscious) ideation. J Abnorm Psychol 3:33-42, 1909

18. Rosenbaum M: The role of the term schizophrenia in the decline of diagnoses of multiple personality. Arch Gen Psychiatry 37:1383-1385, 1980

19. Braun BG: Hypnosis creates multiple personality: myth or reality? Int J Clin Exp Hypn 32:191-197, 1984

20. Kluft RP: Varieties of hypnotic interventions in the treatment of multiple personality. Am J Clin Hypn 24:230-240, 1982

21. Hull CL: Hypnosis and Suggestibility. New York, Appleton-Century, 1933

22. Messerschmidt R: A quantitative investigation of the alleged independent operation of conscious and unconscious processes. J Abnorm Psychol 22: 325-340, 1927

23. White RW, Shevach BJ: Hypnosis and the concept of dissociation. J Abnorm Psychol 37:309-328

24. Taylor WS, Martin MF: Multiple personality. Journal of Abnormal and Social Psychology 39:281-300, 1944

25. American Psychiatric Association: Diagnostic and Statistical Manual of Mental Disorders (First Edition). Washington, DC, American Psychiatric Association, 1952

26. American Psychiatric Association: Diagnostic and Statistical Manual

of Mental Disorders (Second Edition). Washington, DC, American Psychiatric Association, 1968

27. Thigpen CH, Cleckley H: A case of multiple personality. Journal of Abnormal and Social Psychology 49:135-151, 1954

28. Hilgard EH: Hypnotic Susceptibility. New York, Harcourt, Brace, and World, Inc., 1965

29. Allison RB: Diagnosis and Treatment of a Multiple Personality. Davis, California, Private printing, 1977

30. Bliss EL: Multiple personalities: a report of 14 cases with implications for schizophrenia and hysteria. Arch Gen Psychiatry 37:1388-1397, 1980

31. Kluft RP: Hypnotherapeutic crisis intervention in multiple personality. Am J Clin Hypn 26:73-83, 1983

32. Orne MT: The construct of hypnosis: implications of the definition for research and practice. Ann NY Acad Sci 296:14-33, 1977

33. Tellegen A: On measures and conceptions of hypnosis. Am J Clin Hypn 21:219-236, 1979

34. Spanos NP, Barber TX: Toward a congruence in hypnosis research. American Psychologist 29:500-511, 1974

35. Sarbin TR, Coe WC: Hypnosis: A Social Psychological Analysis of Influence Communication. New York, Holt, Rinehart, and Winston, 1972

36. Morgan AH, Johnson DL, Hilgard ER: The stability of hypnotic susceptibility: a longitudinal study. Int J Clin Exp Hypn 22:249-257, 1974

37. Stern DB, Spiegel D, Nee JC: The hypnotic induction profile: normative observations, reliability, and validity. Am J Clin Hypn 21:219-236, 1979

38. Katz NW: Comparative efficacy of behavioral training, training plus relaxation, and a sleep/trance hypnotic induction in increasing hypnotic susceptibility. J Consult Clin Psychol 47:119-127, 1979

39. Frischholz EJ, Blumstein R, and Spiegel D: Comparative efficacity of hypnotic behavioral training and sleep/trance hypnotic induction: comment on Katz. J Consult Clin Psychol 50:766-769, 1982

40. Perry C: Is hypnotizability modifiable? Int J Clin Exp Hypn 25:125-146, 1977

41. Barber J: Hypnosis and the unhypnotizable. Am J Clin Hypn 23: 4-7, 1980

42. Shafer DW, Hernandez A: Hypnosis, pain, and the context of therapy. Int J Clin Exp Hypn 26:143-153, 1978

43. Frischholz EJ, Spiegel D: Hypnosis is not therapy. Bulletin of the British Society of Experimental and Clinical Hypnosis 6:3-8, 1983

44. Gibson HB: A comment on Frischholz and Spiegel's "Hypnosis is not therapy." Bulletin of the British Society of Experimental and Clinical Hypnosis 6:9-13, 1983

45. Vingoe FJ: A comment on Frischholz and Spiegel's "Hypnosis is not therapy" Bulletin of the British Society of Experimental and Clinical Hypnosis 6:15-18, 1983

46. McCue PA: A comment on Frischholz and Spiegel's "Hypnosis is not therapy." Bulletin of the British Society of Experimental and Clinical Hypnosis 6:19-21, 1983

47. Frischholz EJ, Spiegel D: A reply to the comments of Gibson, Vingoe, and McCue. Bulletin of the British Society of Experimental and Clinical Hypnosis 6:23-27, 1983

48. Horowitz SL: Strategies within hypnosis for reducing phobic behavior. J Abnorm Psychol 75:104-112, 1970

49. Spiegel D, Frischholz EJ, Maruffi BL, et al: Hypnotic responsivity and the treatment of flying phobia. Am J Clin Hypn 23:239-247, 1981

50. Morgan AH: The heritability of hypnotic susceptibility in twins. J Abnorm Psychol 82:55-61, 1973

51. Tellegen A, Atkinson G: Openness to absorbing and self-altering experiences ("absorption"), a trait related to hypnotic susceptibility. J Abnorm Psychol 83:268-277, 1974

52. Weitzenhoffer AM, Hilgard ER: Stanford Hypnotic Susceptibility Scale: Form C. Palo Alto, California, Consulting Psychologists Press, 1959

53. Weitzenhoffer AM: Hypnotic susceptibility revisited. Am J Clin Hypn 22: 130-146, 1980

54. Bowers KS: Do the Stanford scales tap the "classic suggestion effect"? Int J Clin Exp Hypn 29:42-53, 1981

55. Weitzenhoffer AM, Hilgard ER: Stanford Hypnotic Susceptibility Scale: Forms A and B. Palo Alto, California, Consulting Psychologists Press, 1959

56. Hilgard ER: The hidden observer and multiple personality. International Journal of Clinical and Experimental Hypnosis 32:248-253, 1984

57. Spanos NP, Hewitt EC: The hidden observer in hypnotic analgesia: discovery or experimental creation? Journal of Personality and Social Psychology 39:1201-1214, 1980

58. Laurence J-R, Perry C: The "hidden observer" phenomenon in hypnosis: Some additional findings. Journal of Abnormal Psychology 90:334-344, 1981

59. Nogrady H, McConkey KM, Laurence J-R, et al: Dissociation, duality, and demand characteristics in hypnosis. J Abnorm Psychol 92:223-235, 1983

60. Bliss EL: Spontaneous self-hypnosis in multiple personality disorder. Psychiatr Clin North Am 7:135-148, 1984

61. Frischholz EJ, Lipman LS, Braun BG: Hypnotizability and multiple

personality disorders. Paper presented at the First International Conference on Multiple Personality/Dissociative States. Chicago, September, 1984

62. Kluft RP: Age regression in multiple personality patients before and after integration. Paper presented at the Annual Meeting of the Society for Clinical and Experimental Hypnosis. San Antonio, October, 1984

6

The Transgenerational Incidence of Dissociation and Multiple Personality Disorder: A Preliminary Report

Bennett G. Braun, M.D., M.S.

6

The Transgenerational Incidence of Dissociation and Multiple Personality Disorder: A Preliminary Report

The past 10 years has been a time of renewed interest in the dissociative disorders from both a theoretical (1, 2) and a clinical (3) perspective. In a very short time, a substantial literature has amassed (4). One of the driving forces behind this increase in attention has been the recognition that dissociative disorders are clinical syndromes distinct from the hysterical neuroses, and the acknowledgement of that recognition in the classification system of the current Diagnostic and Statistical Manual of Mental Disorders, Third Edition (DSM-III) (5). Among these conditions, multiple personality disorder, which has also become the object of intense lay interest and media exposure, has stimulated the greatest amount of recent theoretical exploration and empirical investigation. For example, in addition to the contributions catalogued by Boor and Coons (4), four professional journals have recently devoted special issues to promoting a greater understanding of multiple personality disorder (*American Journal of Clinical Hypnosis*, 26:2, 1983; *Psychiatric Annals*, 14:1, 1984; *Psychiatric Clinics of North America*, 7:1, 1984; *The International Journal of Clinical and Experimental Hypnosis*, 32:2, 1984). In addition, the

The author would like to acknowledge the assistance of Edward J. Frischholz, M.A., Richard P. Kluft, M.D., Ph.D., and Roberta B. Sachs, Ph.D., for their assistance in the preparation of this chapter.

First International Conference on Multiple Personality/Dissociative States was held in Chicago in September 1984.

This proliferation of materials on multiple personality disorder has stimulated new ideas about the causes, diagnosis, and course of the dissociative disorders. Unfortunately, as Greaves notes, much of this thinking has been based on and expressed in single case studies of multiple personality disorder (6); these reports have given little attention to the other dissociative syndromes per se. More recently, some investigators and practitioners have begun to collect systematic observations on large numbers of multiple personality disorder patients (3, 7, 8). A number of specialized programs have begun that are assessing, following, and studying cohorts of individuals suffering multiple personality disorder.

Some reports have suggested that hypnotizability is a personality trait common to dissociative disorders. These reports have further suggested that the interaction of hypnotizability, described by Hilgard (2) and Spiegel and Spiegel (9), with experiences of repeated early child abuse or exposure to traumatic events, constitutes the usual pattern of predisposing factors for the development of multiple personality disorder (3, 10–12; Chapter 3 of this monograph). Other reports describe the transgenerational incidence of child abuse (13, 14). It seems plausible that a population of patients suffering a syndrome associated with child abuse (a phenomenon itself known to have a transgenerational incidence) might have, among close family members, other individuals also suffering the same or a closely related dissociative disorder.

The present study examines the transgenerational incidence of dissociative disorders in a nonconsecutive series of multiple personality disorder patients. It addresses questions about both the genetic and environmental determinants of dissociative phenomena. While this investigation, a preliminary attempt, admittedly lacks the scientific controls appropriate to a definitive exploration, it does permit a liberal test of the null hypothesis of no association. If there were no relationship between the diagnosis of multiple personality disorder and the incidence of dissociative phenomena in the family background of each patient, this should be evident from a simple inspection of the family history.

The following section is a brief discussion of the phenomenon of multiple personality disorder and its classification as a dissociative disorder. Next, data is presented that have emerged from a thorough review of the charts of 18 multiple personality disorder patients. For these patients, sufficiently extensive background information was available to permit an investigator to make a probabilistic diagnosis of the presence or absence of dissociative disorders in the family's other members. This is followed by a critical evaluation of the import of these observations for understanding the nature of dissociative phenomena.

THE PHENOMENON OF MULTIPLE PERSONALITY DISORDER

Multiple personality disorder is one of four dissociative syndromes listed in the current DSM-III (5). The common clinical feature of all dissociative disorders is a temporary (that is, reversible) alteration in the normal integrative functions of consciousness. This alteration is usually characterized by an amnesia for important personal events (that is, psychogenic amnesia) or the lack of recall of one's sense of personal identity (that is, psychogenic fugue, depersonalization disorders, and multiple personality disorder). This chapter will be confined to the phenomena of multiple personality disorder.

Most current investigators agree that although the symptoms of multiple personality disorder were reported sporadically prior to the 19th century and described in many 19th century accounts that stimulated considerable interest, it was the famous cases reported by Janet (15) and Prince (16) that brought the disorder worldwide recognition. This recognition, however, was short-lived (approximately 25 years) for two reasons. First, the introduction and wide acceptance of the term "schizophrenia" by Bleuler may have promoted the misdiagnosis of multiple personality disorder symptoms as schizophrenia (17). To this day, the overlap of some symptoms shared by schizophrenia and multiple personality disorder (such as hallucinated voices) can prove misleading. Second, many early practitioners began to regard multiple personality disorder as the end product of "hypnotic suggestion." The consequence of this view was that multiple personality disorder was not considered to be a genuine diagnostic entity worthy of scientific investigation. Many clinicians still react to the diagnosis of multiple personality disorder with skepticism.

The possibility that many multiple personality disorder patients were incorrectly diagnosed as suffering from another psychiatric disorder is given credence and support by workers who studied a large consecutive series of multiple personality disorder patients (18). They found that for 100 multiple personality disorder patients, drawn from nearly as many referral sources, an average of 6.8 years had elapsed between a patient's initial mental health assessment and the rendering of the correct diagnosis. The range of diagnoses that these patients received, however, was not limited to schizophrenia; it reflected the entire range of psychiatric disorders.

Recent studies by Kampman have been said to demonstrate the hypnotic production of "multiple personalities" (19) and to show thereby that multiple personality disorder is the iatrogenic consequence of hypnotic suggestion. However, several workers have offered arguments that such a reading speciously over-extends the data of the Kampman study and vitiates its genuine contribution (10, 20). These clinicians independently noted that hypnotically created multiple personalities have no life history of their own, show no psychophysiological involvement when reliving the memories of past events, and do not give reports that can be objectively corroborated by external sources. None of those "hypnotically created" multiple personality disorder cases bears a close relation to multiple personality disorder as it is observed clinically (10, 20). Kluft (10) has pointed out that several phenomena can be elicited under hypnosis and misinterpreted as multiple personality disorder. He cautions against assuming that such entities are manifestations of multiple personality disorder, and acknowledges that clinicians without experience may encounter difficulties in making the distinction. In addition, it has been established that the symptoms of multiple personality disorder have been observed in patients who have never before been hypnotized (10, 20). These considerations severely mitigate the criticism that multiple personality disorder is not a genuine diagnostic entity because it is an artifact of hypnotic suggestion.

Many contemporary theorists have proposed that multiple personality disorder, although not the end product of hypnotic suggestion, is most likely to develop in persons who are highly hypnotizable (1, 3, 7, 9, 10, 20, 21). Two recent studies support the contention that multiple personality disorder patients are significantly more hypnotizable than other clinical groups (22, 23). These reports raise further questions about the relation between hypnotizability and dissociation, an issue discussed by Frischholz in Chapter 5 of this monograph.

In the past, multiple personality disorder has been regarded as a rare condition with infrequent incidence. A 1944 review of the literature reported only 76 documented cases of the disorder (24). However, as noted earlier, it is almost impossible to estimate the incidence or prevalence of this syndrome with accuracy, because many multiple personality disorder patients have been incorrectly diagnosed (18, 25). Furthermore, many multiple personality disorder patients appear capable of functioning adaptively in their everyday lives over long periods of time. In these individuals there is usually no apparent gross deficit in functioning. In addition, most multiple personality disorder patients hide their disorder and initially present with symptoms of a more common problem, most often depression (18, 25).

The classification of multiple personality disorder as a dissociative disorder in the current DSM-III (5) marked a new beginning for contemporary scientific efforts to identify this syndrome reliably. While there is debate about the diagnostic criteria per se, there is agreement that they lend themselves well enough to use for research purposes. However, the majority of papers on multiple personality disorder that have appeared since DSM-III have focused on treatment issues. Few have concentrated on understanding the causes and course of this disorder (see Chapter 3 of this monograph). It is typical of this trend, but ironic, that a major etiological theory was advanced in the introduction to an article on therapy results (3). This chapter focuses on the transgenerational incidence of dissociative disorders in the family histories of

18 multiple personality disorder patients. It is hoped that this preliminary attempt will stimulate interest in studying the genetic and environmental determinants of multiple personality disorder.

The Method

The information to be reported below was first collected in the course of taking comprehensive routine clinical histories. Initially, no attempt was made to systematize the gathering of data bearing on dissociation within patients' families because the potential importance of this information was not appreciated. After several cases revealed similar information, I began to suspect the possible existence of transgenerational multiple personality disorder. At that point, a detailed review was made of each patient's chart, and clear patterns were discerned. Subsequent cases were analyzed more carefully in order to substantiate or disconfirm the initial observations. The data reported below are based on 18 nonconsecutive multiple personality disorder patients who were interviewed by me personally. In almost all cases, other family members of the multiple personality disorder patient were interviewed personally, either by me or by one of my colleagues. These cases were selected from a larger pool of consecutive multiple personality disorder cases because extensive family background information was available. The demographic characteristics and referral sources of these 18 patients, meeting DSM-III criteria for multiple personality disorder, are presented in Table 1.

Most of these patients were female (89 percent) and first consulted me before they were 45 years of age (89 percent). The patients came from a wide variety of referral sources. All satisfied DSM-III criteria augmented with the additional criterion of consistency of observed symptoms over time. In almost all cases (94 percent), the symptoms of multiple personality disorder were confirmed as existing by another family member or professional before I made or confirmed the diagnosis of multiple personality disorder.

Several procedures were used to facilitate and clarify the presen-

Table 1. Demographic Information for 18 Multiple Personality Disorder (MPD) Patients

Case Number	Referral Source	Diagnostic Criteria	Confirmation of DSM-III MPD Behavior Before Therapy	Age	Sex	Education	Marital Status	Only Child	Living with Family of Origin after Age 18
1	Telephone Directory	DSM-III	Yes	26	F	College (4 years)	Married	No	After age 18 Yes
2	Therapist	DSM-III	Yes	26	F	College (3 years)	Single	No	Fluctuated
3	Therapist	DSM-III	Yes	31	F	High School	Married	No	No
4	Therapist	DSM-III	Yes	30	F	High School	Married	Yes	No
5	Self-Referred	DSM-III	Yes	35	F	College (2 years)	Single	No	Fluctuated
6	Therapist	DSM-III	Yes	21	F	College (1 year)	Single	No	Yes
7	Telephone Directory	DSM-III	Yes	28	F	College (1 year)	Married	No	Fluctuated
8	Husband	DSM-III	Yes	32	F	Graduate School	Married	No	Yes

9	Friend	DSM-III	Yes	34	F	College (2 years)	Divorced	No	After age 18 Fluctuated
10	Daughter	DSM-III	No	50	F	High School	Divorced	No	Yes
11	Social Service Agency	DSM-III	Yes	30	F	College (2 years)	Married	No	Yes
12	Husband	DSM-III	Yes	48	F	High School	Married	No	No
13	Court	DSM-III	Yes	22	M	High School	Married	No	Yes
14	Newspaper	DSM-III	Yes	44	M	College (4 years)	Married	Yes	Fluctuated
15	Another Patient	DSM-III	Yes	19	F	High School (3 years)	Single	No	No
16	Therapist	DSM-III	Yes	24	F	College (4 years)	Single	No	Adopted at birth and Yes after age 18
17	Therapist	DSM-III	Yes	36	F	Medical School (4 years)	Married	No	Yes
18	Therapist	DSM-III	Yes	33	F	High School	Single	No	No

tation of the data. First, a family background form (FBF) was developed, which focused on five different areas of the family history. These five areas included: 1) the current family environment of the patient; 2) the biological or adopted parents of the patient; 3) the siblings of the patient; 4) the maternal relatives of the patient; and 5) the paternal relatives of the patient. Next, a thorough chart review of each patient's file was conducted and the relevant information was summarized on the FBF. Whenever sufficient information was available, a probabilistic diagnosis (as described below) was given to each relative in the family constellation. This diagnostic procedure focused on: 1) whether there was any evidence of a dissociative disorder, and 2) the particular type of dissociative disorder observed.

Three classes of dissociative disorders were identified. These included: 1) multiple personality disorder (MPD) according to DSM-III criteria; 2) documented psychogenic fugue states (FS) according to DSM-III criteria; and 3) dissociative episodes (DE). The criteria for the category of dissociative episodes were: 1) the individual reports blackouts or missing periods of time; 2) the individual reports finding himself or herself in a place with no idea of how he or she got there; and 3) neither criteria 1 nor 2 is due to another organized mental or neurological disorder and/or alcohol or drug consumption. The use of the DE category permits the probabilistic designation of a dissociative diathesis by history, without implicitly equating this diathesis to any diagnostic entity in DSM-III.

In order to further classify the accuracy of the diagnoses given to other family members, a four point diagnostic certainty scale was developed. A low rating on this scale indicates less diagnostic certainty or corroborative evidence, while higher ratings indicate greater diagnostic confidence. The four anchor points on the diagnostic certainty were as follows: 1–Possible, 2–Probable, 3–Highly Probable, 4–Confirmed (see Table 2 for operational definitions of these ratings.)

The diagnostic certainty rating has two noteworthy features. First, the ratings conform to a Guttman scaling procedure (26) in which higher ratings are assumed to include all of the criteria

Table 2. Rating of Diagnostic Certainty

Rating		Diagnostic Confidence Level
1	Possible Evidence of Dissociation/MPD	The diagnosis is based on consistent historical information provided by the patient on more than one occasion. However, the family member being diagnosed is never observed by a trained professional while manifesting relevant behaviors. No corroborating evidence exists.
2	Probable Evidence of Dissociation/MPD	The criteria for a certainty rating of 1 are fully satisfied. In addition, the patient's report is further corroborated by either: a) the consistent report of another family member; or b) the documentation by a trained mental health professional of dissociative/MPD symptoms that fell short of fulfilling recognized DSM-III criteria.
3	Highly Probable Evidence of Dissociation/MPD	The criteria for a certainty rating of 2 are fully satisfied. In addition, this evidence is further corroborated by either: a) the consistent report of another family member (total of two reports in addition to the patient's); or b) the documentation and full recognition of dissociative/MPD symptoms by a trained mental health professional, but the family member is only seen on a single occasion.
4	Confirmed Evidence of Dissociation/MPD	The criteria for a diagnostic certainty rating of 3 are fully satisfied. In addition, the author or another trained mental health professional personally observed and documented signs of dissociation/MPD in the family member on more than one occasion.

necessary for lower ratings. Second, the ratings emphasize the importance of consistent observation of dissociation/multiple personality disorder over time. In this sense, the present "confirmed" criteria are more stringent than those found in DSM-III.

The use of both a qualitative and quantitative diagnostic system parallels the multiaxial approach used in DSM-III. In an attempt to give a more valid description of the syndrome as observed, data are presented as observations, qualified by the amount and/or nature of available corroborative evidence.

In summary, the method used in this report is a retrospective analysis of a nonconsecutive series of cases. These cases were selected on the basis of the completeness of available family history data. This information was collected routinely rather than systematically. No attempt was made to include a control group or to compare the familial incidence of dissociative disorders with any other clinical disorder.

Despite the data's limitations, they do permit a liberal test of the null hypothesis (that is, there is no transgenerational incidence of dissociation/multiple personality disorder). However, if the null hypothesis is rejected, this data allows no way to determine whether this is due to the selectivity of the sample, the lack of a standardized data collection procedure, or to the lack of an appropriate control or comparison group. These considerations will be addressed in future research.

RESULTS

Observations bearing upon the transgenerational incidence of dissociation/multiple personality disorder in each of the 18 cases studied is presented in Table 3. The case numbers in Table 3 correspond to the case numbers in Table 1.

The data in Table 3 have been organized into five family areas corresponding to those in the FBF. These are: 1) the current family environment of the patient (including spouse/lover, children, or any other person residing in the household); 2) the biological or adoptive parents of the patient; 3) the siblings of the patient (and their offspring); 4) the maternal relatives of the patient; and 5) the paternal relatives of the patient. Both the qualitative diagnosis and diagnostic certainty level for this diagnosis are presented for each family member identified in the Table. The symbol N/A was used whenever information about a particular family area was not available. For reasons of space, Table 3 does not include information on any family member for whom no diagnosis of dissociative disorder was made.

The data reported in Table 3 indicate that there is evidence of dissociation and/or multiple personality disorder in the family histories of the 18 multiple personality disorder patients. An

Table 3. Transgenerational Incidence of Dissociative Disorders (With Diagnostic Certainty Ratings) in the Families of Multiple Personality Disorder (MPD) Patients[1]

Case Number	Current Family	Parents	Siblings	Maternal Relations	Paternal Relations
1	—	Mother (MPD,4) Father (MPD,1)	Brother #1 (DE,1) Brother #2 (DE,1)	Maternal grandmother (MPD,1)	N/A
2	Single	Mother (MPD,4) Father (MPD,2; also had previous diagnosis of FS,4)	Brother (MPD,3) Sister (MPD,1; DE,4) Daughter of Sister (MPD,4)	Grandmother (MPD,2) Grandfather (MPD,2)	Grandfather (MPD,2)
3	Husband (DE,4) Daughter (MPD,4)	Mother (MPD,1) Father (MPD,1)	N/A	N/A	N/A
4	Husband (DE,4) Son #1 (MPD,1) Son #2 (MPD,1)	Mother (MPD,3)	N/A	N/A	N/A
5	Daughter (MPD,2) Live-in Babysitter (MPD,4) Babysitter's Daughter (MPD,2)	Mother (MPD,4)	—	Uncle #1 (MPD,1) Uncle #2 (MPD,1) Uncle #3 (MPD,1) Cousin #1 (MPD,1) Cousin #2 (MPD,1)	N/A

Table 3. *Continued.*

Case Number	Current Family	Parents	Siblings	Maternal Relations	Paternal Relations
6	—	Mother (MPD,4)	Sister #1 (MPD,4)	N/A	N/A
			Sister #2 (MPD,4)		
			Sister #3 (DE,4)		
7	Husband (MPD,2) Son (MPD,2)	Mother (MPD,3) Father (MPD,3)	Brother (MPD,1)	N/A	N/A
8	Husband (DE,2) Daughter (MPD,3)	Mother (MPD,3)	N/A	N/A	N/A
9	Ex-husband (MPD,4)	Mother (MPD,3) Father (MPD,2) Daughter of Brother #1 (DE,1) Son of Brother #1 (MPD,1)	Brother #1 (MPD,3) Brother #2 (DE,2)	Maternal grandmother (MPD,1) Maternal grandfather (DE,1)	N/A
10	Ex-husband #1 (MPD,1) Ex-husband #2 (MPD,3)	N/A	Brother (DE,1)	N/A	N/A
11	Ex-husband (MPD,3) Step-daughter (DE,4)	Mother (MPD,3)	Sister (DE,2)	N/A	N/A

Table 3. Continued.

Case Number	Current Family	Parents	Siblings	Maternal Relations	Paternal Relations
12	Husband (DE,4) Daughter (MPD,1)	Mother (MPD,2) Father (MPD,1)	Brother (MPD,3)	N/A	N/A
13	—	Father (MPD,3) Mother (DE,3)	Brother (DE,1)	N/A	Grandmother (MPD,3)
14	Wife (DE,4) Daughter (MPD,4)	Mother (MPD,3)	Sisters (MPD,3)	N/A	N/A
15	Daughter (MPD,2)	N/A	N/A	N/A	N/A

See Case #5: The Patient is #5's live-in Babysitter.

Case Number	Current Family	Parents	Siblings	Maternal Relations	Paternal Relations
16	Single	Adoptive Mother (MPD,4) Adoptive Father (MPD,1)	Adopted Brother #1 (MPD,1) Adopted Brother #2 (DE,1)	N/A	N/A
17	Husband (DE,3) Daughter (MPD,4)	Mother (MPD,2) Father (MPD,1)	N/A	N/A	N/A
18	Single	Mother (MPD,1) Father (MPD,1)	N/A	N/A	—

[1]For reasons of space, family members for whom no diagnosis was made have not been included.

average of 4.61 family members per patient (SD = 1.92, range = 1–9) showed some evidence of dissociative phenomena. When consideration is restricted to those parents whose diagnoses were assigned a certainty level of 3 or 4, an incidence of multiple personality disorder is observed in the family history of 12 out of 18 multiple personality disorder cases (67 percent). As an illustration of the data underlying this generalization, five of the 18 multiple personality disorder index cases (27.8 percent) had mothers or stepmothers given the diagnosis of multiple personality disorder at a certainty level of 4.

These findings clearly support the hypothesis of the transgenerational incidence of dissociation or multiple personality disorder. Some corroboration can be found in the work of Kluft, who found multiple personality disorder in one or both parents of 40 percent of his childhood multiple personality disorder cases (11), and describes, in passing, a witnessed episode of psychogenic amnesia in one patient's sibling (27).

In order to illustrate how the information in Table 3 was collected and what it may imply, two case examples will be described briefly. In these descriptions, the focus will be on the diagnoses of both the patients and their family members. Information about treatment and outcome issues will not be presented here. The numbers of the case examples correspond to the case numbers in Tables 1 and 3. The reader should be aware that, for reasons of space, these presentations are cursory, omitting most of the data that led to the author's conclusions. Otherwise, each inference drawn would require a separate case report as background.

Case 2

Case 2 was a 26-year-old woman who was referred to me by a colleague. She presented for treatment suffering from anxiety and depression. Therapy was begun, directed toward alleviating her chief complaints. After approximately four months of treatment, I observed signs that led me to consider the possibility of fugue states; I also noted that the diagnosis of multiple personality disorder had to be ruled out. The diagnosis of multiple personality disorder was confirmed 2½ years later. The major reason for this delay in correct diagnosis relates to what Kluft has called the sociology of psychiatric diagnosis and epidemiology (28): during the early 1970s, the incidence of multiple personality disorder was assumed to be very rare, and I assumed my suspicions were inaccurate.

During the period of almost three years before the diagnosis of multiple personality disorder was finally made, the patient repeatedly switched personalities in front of me; at the time, I did not fully recognize these signs for what they were. After three years, I documented a number of signs characteristic of multiple personality disorder. I brought an audiotape of the patient to a senior colleague, who confirmed my suspicions regarding the diagnosis of multiple personality disorder.

Throughout the course of the patient's treatment, I collected extensive family history data and personally interviewed several family members (for example, I interviewed the patient's parents twice). During these sessions, the father was found to have had a history of fugue states during his military service. Consistent reports of his behaviors given by both the patient and her sister suggested a diagnosis of multiple personality disorder. However, I did not personally witness any signs of multiple personality disorder. Consequently, the diagnostic certainty level for this diagnosis (according to the criteria presented earlier) was assessed as 2.

The patient's mother showed obvious classical signs of multiple personality disorder during both interviews. Because I directly observed these signs on two separate occasions, the diagnosis of multiple personality disorder was considered confirmed. Confidence in this diagnosis was further strengthened by consistent descriptions of the mother's multiple personality disorder behaviors given by the patient, her sister, and her niece, who was living with the patient's mother at the time.

The patient referred her sister to me for treatment of anxiety and depression following the sister's recent divorce. I saw the patient's sister for approximately 1½ years. During this period, I witnessed several of the sister's dissociative episodes. In addition, the history given by the sister's daughter also indicated a history of dissociation (certainty level = 4). Information provided by the patient indicated a diagnosis of multiple personality disorder (certainty level = 1). I could not confirm a diagnosis of multiple personality disorder for the patient's sister. However, the patient's sister also referred her daughter to me for treatment of school problems. According to the predictor indices provided by Kluft (11), the daughter would be highly suspect for childhood multiple personality disorder with a diagnostic certainty level of 4.

Consistent reports from the patient, her parents, and her sister suggested that the patient's brother also suffered from multiple personality disorder (certainty level = 3). However, there is no record of a trained professional observing his behavior. An interesting incident regarding the brother occurred during an interview with the parents. I began asking the parents questions about the brother based on information given by the patient and her sister. The mother repeatedly tried to deny her daughters' reports, but the father looked at her and offered observations and described events that confirmed these reports. The mother then reluctantly admitted that some of the things said about the brother might be possible. This illustrates the "rule of secrecy" that characterizes the family of multiple personality disorder patients (12). The mother's initial denial of her son's behavior was an unsuccessful attempt to present the family as "normal."

Based on the consistent reports of the patient and her sister, both of the maternal grandparents showed signs of multiple personality disorder (certainty level = 2). Information from the patient and her sister consistently suggests that the paternal grandfather suffered from multiple personality disorder (certainty level = 2). The patient received her consistent love and protection from her paternal grandmother, who evidenced no history of multiple personality disorder symptoms or dissociation. These data show probable multiple personality disorder in four generations.

Case 13

Case 13 is a 22-year-old married male who was referred by the Court for a diagnostic evaluation. The possibility of multiple personality disorder had been considered by those making the referral. This individual was being tried for his father's murder. In giving his history, he reported that his father was a pharmacist who was viewed by others as a "pillar of the community." However, he said that his father also was involved in dealing drugs, and had organized crime connections. The patient admitted that he was a "runner" in his father's drug operation. He also stated that his father was significantly in debt and had asked his son to kill him so that the life insurance money could be used to pay his debts. The father believed that suicide would negate payment of the policy. This information was confirmed by other individuals, as well. The patient could not bring himself to kill his father. He recruited another person to commit the actual murder. This person confirmed the wish to be murdered with the father, and did commit the murder several weeks later. Both the patient and the actual murderer were arrested by the police and placed on trial.

I saw the patient daily over a week's time. During this period, the diagnosis of multiple personality disorder was confirmed (certainty level = 4), and I personally witnessed body, face, voice, and attitude changes. Additional interviews with two of the patients' brothers, his sister, his wife, cousins, and neighbors confirmed behavior changes characteristic of multiple personality disorder.

Based on reports from the patient, his wife, his family, and neighbors, the father was a highly probable multiple personality disorder (certainty level = 3). He was described as an unpredictable man who displayed inappropriate anger and had a history of observed voice and behavioral changes. Both his family and the patient said that the father acted as if "he were two separate people." These reports, along with the patient's claim that his father was both a "drug dealer" and a "pillar of the community," are consistent with a diagnosis of multiple personality disorder.

Information collected from the patient, his wife, and his siblings suggested that the patient's mother, who had since died, had a history of dissociative episodes (certainty level = 3). All sources noted that, at times, she would stare blankly into space. She was quite changeable; her affect was described as labile. The mother was also described as an hysteric. This woman, who was usually confined to a wheelchair, had evidenced inexplicable periods of improved motor coordination.

Data provided by the patient, his family, and his wife also suggest that his paternal grandmother is suffering from multiple personality disorder (certainty level = 3). She was consistently described as "unpredictable," "changeable," and troubled by "memory difficulties." Collectively, her family characterized her as a "terror" because of her inappropriate screaming and uncontrolled behavior. In addition, her behavior toward her children was erratic. She had a history of physically abusing them, but from time to time she showered them with loving affection. This illustrates the history of inconsistent love and abuse that is so frequently reported in families of multiple personality disorder patients (29).

There appeared to be little evidence of a discrete dissociative disorder in any of the patient's siblings. The sole possible exception was one brother's reporting a history of dissociative episodes. Many of these episodes were clearly related to periods of alcohol consumption. However, the brother reported one blackout that occurred when he had not been drinking; he found himself somewhere, having no recollection of how he got there.

The patient was ultimately found guilty of manslaughter. He was sentenced to 25 years in prison. The jury did not appear to acknowledge the psychiatric evidence offered by the defense and did not deliberate over the issue of mitigating circumstances due to a mental disorder.

SUMMARY

The data reported in Table 3 support the hypothesis that the incidence of dissociation or multiple personality disorder is transgenerational. Some evidence of dissociative phenomena was reported and/or observed in the family histories of all 18 multiple personality disorder cases. When consideration is restricted to those cases in which the dissociation or multiple personality disorder was seen by me, repeatedly over time, the presence of these phenomena still was observed in 12 of 18 (67 percent) of the cases. Either figure is sufficient to invalidate the null hypothesis of no association.

What do these findings mean? First, the data support the hypothesis of a transgenerational association. However, several factors preclude a clear interpretation of the mechanism that underlies this connection. One confounding factor is the use of a selected sample chosen on the basis of the availability of information on the patients' family histories. On the one hand, it might be assumed that this prejudices data in favor of confirming an association. On the other hand, however, many multiple personality disorder patients come from families that deny anything problematic has ever occurred, and whose members are unwilling to share any data or come in for interviews. One might speculate (but could not conclude) that there could be either more, less, or the same amount of dissociative pathologies in these other families. Another factor is that the information was collected routinely rather than systematically. Furthermore, the statistical analyses were carried out retrospectively. Future studies on the transgenerational incidence of dissociative phenomena should collect family history data prospectively, in a standardized fashion, on a large consecutive series of patients with confirmed diagnoses of multiple personality disorder or other dissociative disorders.

Future work must also identify what types of control and/or comparison groups would be most appropriate for the comparative assessment of the transgenerational rate of incidence of dissociative phenomena with the transgenerational rate of incidence of other psychiatric disorders.

The data presented in this report also raise questions about the relative influence of genetic and environmental factors in the development of a dissociative disorder. These questions cannot be resolved without extensive, well controlled, anterospective studies. It is hoped that the twin study paradigms that have proven so illuminating in appreciating familial factors in schizophrenia will become applicable in the study of dissociative disorders, as well. Dr. Roberta Sachs and I have offered a plausible, tentative explanation of the way genetic and environmental variables may interact in the development of multiple personality disorder in Chapter 3 of this monograph.

In conclusion, the data reported indicate that the incidence of dissociation and multiple personality disorder is transgenerational. Some evidence of dissociation or multiple personality disorder was observed in the family histories of the cases studied. Future research needs to identify the mechanism that underlies this transgenerational association.

References

1. Braun BG: Towards a theory of multiple personality and other dissociative phenomena. Psychiatr Clin North Am 7:171-194, 1984

2. Hilgard ER: Divided Consciousness: Multiple Controls in Human Thought and Action. New York, John Wiley and Sons, 1977

3. Kluft RP: Treatment of multiple personality disorder. Psychiatr Clin North Am 7:9-30, 1984

4. Boor M, Coons PM: A comprehensive bibliography of literature pertaining to multiple personality. Psychol Rep 53:295-310, 1983

5. American Psychiatric Association: Diagnostic and Statistical Manual of Mental Disorders (Third Edition). Washington, DC, American Psychiatric Association, 1980

6. Greaves GB: Multiple personality: 165 years after Mary Reynolds. J Nerv Ment Dis 168:577-596, 1980

7. Bliss EL: Multiple personalities: a report of 14 cases with implications for schizophrenia and hysteria. Arch Gen Psychiatry 37:1388-1397, 1980

8. Horevitz RP, Braun BG: Are multiple personalities borderline? Psychiatr Clin North Am 7:69-88, 1984

9. Spiegel H, Spiegel D: Trance and Treatment: Clinical Uses of Hypnosis. New York, Basic Books, 1978

10. Kluft RP: Varieties of hypnotic interventions in the treatment of multiple personality. Am J Clin Hypn 24:230-240, 1982

11. Kluft RP: Multiple personality in childhood. Psychiatr Clin North Am 7:121-134, 1984

12. Braun BG: The role of the family in the development of multiple personality disorder. International Journal of Family Psychiatry (in press)

13. Gil DG: Violence Against Children. Cambridge, Harvard University Press, 1970

14. Justice B, Justice R: The Abusing Family. New York, Human Sciences Press, 1976

15. Janet P: L'Automatisme Psychologique. Paris, Felix Alcan, 1889

16. Prince M: The Dissociation of a Personality. New York, Longmans Green, 1906

17. Rosenbaum M: The role of the term schizophrenia in the decline of diagnoses of multiple personality. Arch Gen Psychiatry 37:1383-1385, 1980

18. Putnam FW, Post RM, Guroff JJ, et al: 100 cases of multiple personality disorder. Presented at the Annual Meeting of the American Psychiatric Association. New Research Abstract #77, New York, 1983

19. Kampman R: Hypnotically induced multiple personality: an experimental study. Int J Clin Exp Hypn 24:215-227, 1976

20. Braun BG: Hypnosis creates multiple personality: myth or reality. Int J Clin Exp Hypn 32:191-197, 1984

21. Braun BG: Uses of hypnosis with multiple personality. Psychiatric Annals 14:34-40, 1984

22. Bliss EL: Multiple personalities, related disorders, and hypnosis. Am J Clin Hypn 26:114-123, 1983

23. Frischholz EJ, Lipman LS, Braun BG: Special hypnotic phenomena and multiple personality disorder. Paper presented at the First International Congress for the Study of Multiple Personality Disorder/ Dissociative States, Chicago, September, 1984

24. Taylor WS, Martin MF: Multiple personality. Journal of Abnormal and Social Psychology 49:281-290, 1944

25. Kluft RP: An introduction to multiple personality. Psychiatric Annals 14:19-24, 1984

26. Guttman L: The basis for scalogram analysis, in Measurement and prediction. Edited by Stouffer SA, Guttman L, Suchman EA, et al. Princeton, N.J., Princeton University Press, 1950

27. Kluft RP: Hypnotherapy of childhood multiple personality disorder. Am J Hypn (in press)

28. Kluft RP: The epidemiology of multiple personality. Paper presented at a course given at the Annual Meeting of American Psychiatric Association, Chicago, May, 1979

29. Sachs RG, Goodwin J, Braun BG: The role of child abuse in the development of multiple personality disorder, in Multiple Personality and Dissociation. Edited by Braun BG, Kluft RP. New York, Guilford Press (in press)

7

Children of Parents with Multiple Personality Disorder

Philip M. Coons, M.D.

7

Children of Parents with Multiple Personality Disorder

A renewal of interest in multiple personality disorder has been evident since the early 1970s. Heralding this renewed interest were the publication of *Sybil* (1) and the first modern scientific study of multiple personality disorder by Ludwig et al. (2). In the 1980s the literature has burgeoned (3), and investigators have broadened our understanding of the disorder's origins (4), psychophysiology (5–7), and familial context (8).

Although the Diagnostic and Statistical Manual of Mental Disorders, Third Edition (DSM-III) suggests that multiple personality disorder is rare (9), this is disputed by some clinicians (4, 10). In fact, no estimates of the incidence of multiple personality disorder were uncovered by my literature review. There were neither estimates available for the incidence of multiple personality disorder in childhood, nor estimates for its incidence within families in which one or both parents are afflicted with multiple personality disorder. Multiple personality disorder is thought to develop during childhood, but is not usually diagnosed until late adolescence or early adulthood (11). The adult form of the syndrome has been adequately described elsewhere (9, 12–16). Physical and sexual abuse during childhood are common in these patients' histories. Putnam et al. found an 83 percent incidence of sexual abuse and a 75 percent incidence of physical abuse in their detailed study of 100 cases (17). Only a few reports have described multiple personality disorder's existence in childhood (11, 18–21)

However, although multiple personality disorder patients themselves have been the subjects of numerous detailed single case studies, usually their children are mentioned only in passing, or in brief allusions. Chris Sizemore, known in the literature as "Eve," has tried to describe the impact of her condition on her daughter (22); but many studies have bypassed the dilemmas of the children of multiple personality disorder parents.

A fairly extensive literature review identified five additional references regarding the children of multiple personality disorder patients. Stoller's patient, Mrs. G., was described in *Splitting: A Case of Female Masculinity* (23). Mrs. G. was a divorced housewife with two teenaged sons. She had craved to be a parent and her sons were the most valued people in her life. Although Stoller mentioned the boys' having "psychopathology," he was vague as to the nature of their difficulties. He did note that one son was trying to protect his mother, who was quite impaired.

Goodwin and Owen (24) described a woman who had been married four times. She had two daughters, aged 14 and 15 years, both of whom had been sexually abused by their stepfather. The mother's five personalities were revealed after she joined a group of mothers who were members of families in which sexual abuse had occurred. It is of interest that she herself had been the victim of incest.

Levinson and Berry (25) described a 38-year-old Spanish-American woman with multiple personality disorder who had two daughters, aged 10 and 17 years, all of whom lived with her and her lesbian lover of nine years. Although the patient and her lover thought the children were unaware of her dissociation, in fact they were quite cognizant of it and actually colluded in encouraging their mother's dissociation. The authors made no observations regarding the emotional health of the daughters.

In a single case report of a divorced 30-year-old Alaskan father with multiple personality disorder, Brown (26) described the complex circumstances that surrounded efforts to intervene on behalf of his 18-month-old daughter, whom he had battered.

There were legal delays, punitive community attitudes, and conflicting psychiatric opinions, all of which hampered the ultimately unsuccessful attempt to obtain protection for the daughter and treatment for the father.

Finally, Kluft (11) described five cases of multiple personality disorder in children; two of these children had parents who themselves suffered multiple personality disorder. Both children had been beaten by one of their affected parents' alternate personalities.

The study presented in this chapter was undertaken because of the current lack of knowledge regarding the children of multiple personality disorder patients. The paucity of data on this subject may become a glaring public health dilemma. An increasing number of multiple personality disorder patients are being identified, most of whom are women with children, or women who are of child-bearing age. Clinicians must contend with the impact of such patients' pathology upon their current and/or projected families (8).

At the start of the present study, the following questions were asked:

1. What is the incidence of emotional illness in the children of parents with multiple personality disorder?
2. What is the cause of emotional illness in the children of parents with multiple personality disorder?
3. What is the incidence of dissociative disorders in children of parents with multiple personality disorder?
4. How often do parents with multiple personality disorder, who were usually abused themselves, abuse their own children?

METHODS

Since 1973, I have followed a series of 20 patients with multiple personality disorder. All patients met the DSM-III criteria for multiple personality (9). In addition, they all had amnesia, which I specifically require as an additional criterion for the diagnosis (13, 14). The patients in this series were matched for age and sex with 20 psychiatric patients whose diagnoses did not include any form

Table 1.   Diagnoses Given to Patients in the Control Group (*N*=20)

A. Primary Diagnoses:	
1. Dysthymic disorder	6
2. Major depression, recurrent	4
3. Borderline personality disorder	3
4. Major depression, single episode	2
5. Bipolar disorder–manic	2
6. Conduct disorder	1
7. Separation-anxiety disorder	1
8. Bulimia	1
B. Secondary and Tertiary Diagnoses	
1. Alcoholism	5
2. Dependent personality disorder	4
3. Histrionic personality disorder	3
4. Drug dependence	3
5. Passive-aggressive personality disorder	2
6. Borderline personality disorder	1
7. Compulsive personality disorder	1
8. Borderline intelligence	1

of dissociative disorder or schizophrenia. Diagnoses of the control group patients are summarized in Table 1.

Detailed psychiatric histories were taken of the patients' children in each group. The children's psychiatric records were examined when they were available. In several instances, the children were interviewed and examined. In addition to checking the emotional health of the children in both groups of patients, the following data was routinely gathered on each patient: detailed psychiatric history; mental status examination; physical examination; social history from relatives or friends; and psychological testing (usually the Minnesota Multiphasic Personality Inventory and either the Wechsler Adult Intelligence Scale or the Shipley-Hartford Intelligence Test). The groups were compared by means of chi-square or Student's *t*-tests, and a probability level of 0.05 was used to determine significance.

RESULTS

Of the 20 patients with multiple personality disorder, 17 (85 percent) were female. The mean age was 29 years, ranging from 14

Table 2. Multiple Personality Disorder Group Compared with Control
Group*

	MPD Group (N=20)	Control Group (N=20)	p Values
Education	11.7 yr	13.0 yr	NS
Intelligence Quotient	101.5	106.7	NS
Marital Status (never married)	4	8	NS
Sexual Abuse Suffered	15	1	$p<.005$
Physical Abuse Suffered	11	1	$p<.005$
Number of Children	23	28	NS
Psychiatric Disturbance in Children	9	1	$p<.005$
Parental Abuse of Children	2	0	NS

*Except where otherwise indicated, figures refer to MPD or control parents.

to 47 years. There were no significant differences between groups
in terms of race, occupation, intelligence, or education. Both
groups were predominately Caucasian and blue-collar. Comparisons are offered on Table 2. The multiple personality disorder
group had a mean education of 11.7 years, and a mean IQ of 101.5.
In terms of marital status, the multiple personality disorder group
had more marriages (22 versus 12) and more divorces (16 versus
eight) than the control group, but these differences did not quite
reach statistical significance. This near-achievement of statistical
significance is deceptive, however. It is skewed because one patient
in the multiple personality disorder group had been married and
divorced five times.

The multiple personality disorder patient group had a total of 23
children, and the control group had a total of 28 children.
Unfortunately, we were unable to control for the numbers,
genders, and ages of children, and for the number of children per
subject. The multiple personality disorder group included 12
patients who had no children; 10 control subjects were childless.
The number of children in the multiple personality disorder
families ranged from one to six per family, and their ages ranged
from four to 31 years. The number of children in the control
families ranged from one to eight per family, and their ages ranged
from six to 23 years.

Of the 20 patients with multiple personality disorder, eight had

Table 3.   Psychiatric Disturbances in Children of Multiple Personality
Disorder Parents*

	Age	Sex	Diagnosis
Case 1	9	Male	Conduct disorder, socialized, aggressive
Case 2	12	Male	Mixed specific developmental disorder
Case 3	4	Male	Atypical dissociative disorder
Case 4	15	Male	Mental retardation, severe
Case 5	10	Male	Conduct disorder, socialized, nonaggressive
Case 6	20	Male	Antisocial personality disorder, mixed substance abuse
Case 7	15	Male	Multiple personality disorder
Case 8	17	Male	Conduct disorder, socialized, nonaggressive
Case 9	22	Female	Passive-aggressive personality disorder

*Note: Cases 1 and 2, Cases 3 and 4, Cases 5 and 6, and Cases 7 and 8 belong to the same
respective sibships.

produced children. Of the 23 children of multiple personality
disorder patients, nine (39 percent) had diagnosed psychiatric
disturbances. These are listed in Table 3. Of the 28 children in the
control group, only one had a diagnosed psychiatric disturbance—
attention deficit disorder in an adopted child. The differences
between these two groups were statistically significant ($\chi^2=7.81$;
$p < .005$).

The incidence of dissociative disorder in this small sample of 23
children was two (nine percent). Interestingly, although there
were 15 male children and eight female children in the series,
only one out of eight (12 percent) of the female children had a
psychiatric disturbance, compared to eight out of 15 (53 percent) of
the male children. Another interesting finding was that eight of
the nine disturbed children came from four families. These four
families were marked by severity in both marital dysfunction and
the pathology of the index patient's multiple personality disorder.

The sample size did not allow running valid correlations
between sibship size and vulnerability. It would be interesting to
see whether increasing sibship sizes augment or dampen the
impact of parental pathology. The sample size did not permit
conclusions to be drawn about the relation between the genders of
the afflicted parents with the genders of the disturbed children. As
an additional consequence of the limited sample size, parallels
could not be found between children's ages and psychopathology.

Naturally, one would expect to find more evidences of pathology with longer follow-up. These are subjects for future research.

In this series of 20 patients with multiple personality disorder, there had been a 55 percent occurrence of physical abuse, a 75 percent occurrence of sexual abuse, and an 85 percent occurrence of abuse of either kind during childhood. In every instance except one, the abuse was perpetrated by fathers, stepfathers, or other male relatives. However, only two of 23 (nine percent) children of multiple personality disorder patients were abused by their multiple personality parent or his or her spouse. One affected mother and her spouse neglected their baby (Case 1). The second was sexually abused by the parent who did not suffer multiple personality disorder (Case 4). Among the controls, one parent had been physically abused (beaten) and one had been sexually abused (fondled by a neighbor). There were no abuses inflicted on the control group's children. All differences between subjects and controls for abuses experienced and abuses endured by their children were significant at the $p < .005$ level.

CASE PRESENTATIONS

Case Example 1

Mrs. A., a 37-year-old woman, twice married and divorced, had been sexually abused during childhood by her father and several other male relatives. She suffered classical multiple personality disorder. Her eldest son, aged 12 years, had been removed from her care by the welfare department when he was six months of age. The grounds for this action were extreme neglect, including starvation. Both the patient and her first husband neglected this child because of their extremely heavy substance abuse and the patient's frequent dissociation. The son's diagnoses included mixed learning disabilities and impaired fine and gross motor control. These disorders were thought to have been caused by the parents' neglect. Her youngest son, aged nine years and fathered by her second husband, was diagnosed as a conduct disturbance, socialized, aggressive type, after he started a fire at school. This child was not known to have ever been neglected. On follow-up, Mrs. A. continues to dissociate and appears to have little motivation for therapy.

Case Example 2

Mrs. B., a 31-year-old divorced woman with three children, had been physically abused by her own father during childhood. She had multiple personality disorder. Her first child, a boy 15 years of age, was the product of an incestuous relationship between Mrs. B. and her brother. He was diagnosed as being severely mentally retarded. A 13-year-old daughter had no psychiatric illness. Mrs. B.'s youngest child, aged four years, was diagnosed as having an atypical dissociative disorder. His symptoms included sleep-walking episodes. His mother addressed him by several different names (including "little man" because of his corporal size). None of these children were known to have been overtly neglected. On follow-up, Mrs. B. continues to dissociate and appears poorly motivated for therapy.

Case Example 3

Mrs. C., a 44-year-old woman, separated, with multiple personality disorder, had been abused sexually by her father during childhood. Of her three children, her youngest, a 10-year-old boy, was diagnosed as having a conduct disturbance, socialized, nonaggressive; and her eldest son, aged 20 years, was diagnosed as having an antisocial personality disorder and mixed substance abuse. None of her children were known to have been abused. Mrs. C. has been in therapy for five years and continues to dissociate.

Case Example 4

Mrs. D. was a 33-year-old twice-married woman with multiple personality disorder that became clinically evident during her first marriage. Her first husband was a physically abusive man who mistreated her harshly. He also abused their second son sexually.

This boy, a 15-year-old, has developed multiple personality disorder as a consequence. Their eldest son, aged 17 years, was diagnosed as suffering from a conduct disorder, socialized, nonaggressive. A 10-year-old daughter had shown no psychiatric disturbance. Mrs. D., like the others, continues to dissociate. She discontinued therapy because of strong secondary gain factors.

DISCUSSION

In this study, the occurrence of psychiatric disturbances in the children of multiple personality disorder parents is high: 39 percent. Due to the preliminary nature of this pilot study, any efforts to offer causal explanations must be understood as tentative and speculative. Since most of the psychiatrically disturbed children were male offspring whose identified multiple personality disorder parents were female, and since the female multiple personality disorder parents usually had been abused by a male relative, one obvious but tentative conclusion is that in some instances, the male children of a female multiple personality disorder parent are at risk for receiving subtle retaliatory abuses that this study could not detect. Anecdotal support for this speculation was recently provided by a pregnant female multiple personality disorder patient, who openly expressed her hopes that her firstborn child would not be a boy. She was painfully aware of her hatred toward men, which arose out of extensive physical and sexual child abuse perpetrated by her father. She feared she might abuse a male child.

Another reason for psychiatric illness in these children might be the severe illness and continuing dissociation in their multiple personality disorder mothers. This is supported by the data in the present study, in which eight of the nine emotionally disturbed children had mothers who continued to dissociate and/or were poorly motivated for therapy. There are other factors that undoubtedly contribute to the psychiatric disturbances of these children, such as psychiatrically disturbed or absent fathers, poor child-rearing practices, and ongoing child abuse. A definitive answer regarding the cause of psychiatric illness in children of multiple personality disorder parents must await further studies.

The occurrence of multiple personality disorder across genera-tions was established by Kluft (11) and is described in numerous other anecdotal reports. In the current study, there was one mother-son pair in which both had multiple personality disorder, and one mother-son pair in which the mother had multiple personality disorder and the son had an atypical dissociative disorder. Thus, two out of 23 children (nine percent) of the multiple personality parents had some form of dissociative disor-der. On the basis of my experience and research, I would agree with Elliott (18) that the occurrence of multiple personality disorder in a child should be considered presumptive evidence of child abuse until proven otherwise. Child protective services should be involved immediately. Although many individuals with multiple personality disorder are exemplary parents, others and/or their paramours or spouses have been known to abuse their children (11, 24, 26).

The patients in this study are in ongoing follow-up. Thus far, the incidence of child abuse encountered in this study (14 percent) is low but significant. It is possible that as more children are born to the patients in this study and as more time passes, the number of abuse cases in this study may rise. Of the two abuse cases recounted here, only one was perpetrated by a multiple personal-ity disorder patient. The other was perpetrated by a father, the spouse of a patient in the study. In neither case was the patient or family in therapy when the abuse occurred. I have generally been impressed by the positive, constructive, and caring attitude that many multiple personality disorder mothers have toward their children. They were abused as children and strive valiantly to protect their children against similar misfortunes.

Clearly, however, there is a need for rapid intervention in families of multiple personality disorder patients if an angry alternate personality or the patient's spouse or paramour abuses or threatens to abuse a child (8). Most states now have laws requiring the clinician to contact a child protective agency if actual abuse occurs, so that the child may be removed from the home on a temporary or permanent basis and placed in a protective setting.

Many areas also have family support centers, where children can be left to give an overwhelmed parent "time-out," before he or she loses control and becomes abusive.

As is often the case, a pilot study of this kind may raise more questions than it answers. Questions deserving of further research include the following:

1. To what extent do children and spouses collude in maintaining the continued dissociation of a multiple personality disorder parent?
2. What can be said of the child-rearing practices of multiple personality disorder parents and their spouses or paramours?
3. What are the responses of children toward their multiple personality disorder parents? Do some become "superkids" despite the disability of their parent? Do some become protective of their ill parent?

The chapters in this monograph indicate a clear need for further education of members of the psychiatric profession about multiple personality disorder. The early recognition of this condition, when it first occurs in childhood, should result in reduced treatment time for the condition per se in those affected children (11), and a reduction in the incidence of child abuse in the families such individuals will create, years later, as parents. The psychiatric profession must move to teach other professionals involved in treating child abuse and incest victims how to recognize multiple personality disorder, and where to refer such patients for treatment. Both this study and the work of Kluft (11) indicate that the children of multiple personality parents are at risk, and should be examined, worked with preventively to minimize future psychiatric morbidity, and treated promptly if they show signs of established or emerging emotional disorders.

SUMMARY

Twenty patients with multiple personality disorder were matched for age (mean age 29) and sex (85 percent female) with 20 nondissociative disordered, nonschizophrenic inpatients. Detailed psychiatric histories were taken concerning their children and, if available, the children's psychiatric records were examined. In several instances the children were examined. Individuals with multiple personality disorder had a greater number of marriages than the control group, although this finding did not quite achieve statistical significance. Although the multiple personality disorder patients had been physically and sexually abused at a very high rate (85 percent), their children have been abused at a much lower rate, thus far (nine percent). The incidence of psychiatric illness in children of patients with multiple personality disorder (39 percent) was statistically significant when compared with the children of patients from the control group (four percent). There was a nine percent incidence of dissociative disorder in the children of patients with multiple personality disorder. The data suggest that although children of parents with multiple personality disorder are susceptible to child abuse, the incidence of child abuse is relatively low, especially if the parent with multiple personality disorder is in therapy. The incidence of psychiatric disorder in children of patients with multiple personality disorder is quite high, and is probably related to a complex set of factors including multiple marriages, dissociation in the multiple personality disorder parents, lack of parenting skills, and psychiatric illness in the multiple personality disorder patient's spouse.

References

1. Schreiber FR: Sybil. Chicago, Henry Regnery, 1973

2. Ludwig AM, Brandsma JM, Wilbur CB, et al: The objective study of a multiple personality, or, are four heads better than one? Arch Gen Psychiatry 26:293-310, 1972

3. Boor M, Coons PM: A comprehensive bibliography of literature pertaining to multiple personality. Psychol Rep 53:295-310, 1983

4. Kluft RP: Treatment of multiple personality disorder. Psychiatr Clin North Am 7:9-29, 1984

5. Braun BG: Neurophysiologic changes in multiple personality due to integration: A preliminary report. Am J Clin Hypn 26:84-92, 1983

6. Braun BG: Psychophysiologic phenomena in multiple personality and hypnosis. Am J Clin Hypn 26:124-137, 1983

7. Putnam FW: The psychophysiologic investigation of multiple personality disorder. Psychiatr Clin North Am 7:31-40, 1984

8. Kluft RP, Braun BG, Sachs R: Multiple personality, intrafamilial abuse, and family psychiatry. International Journal of Family Psychiatry (in press)

9. American Psychiatric Association: Diagnostic and Statistical Manual of Mental Disorders, Third Edition. Washington, DC, American Psychiatric Association, 1980

10. Bliss EL: Spontaneous self-hypnosis in multiple personality disorder. Psychiatr Clin North Am 7:135-148, 1984

11. Kluft RP: Multiple personality disorder in childhood. Psychiatr Clin North Am 7:121-134, 1984

12. Boor M: The multiple personality epidemic: additional cases and inferences regarding diagnosis, etiology, dynamics, and treatment. J Nerv Ment Dis 170:302-304, 1982

13. Coons PM: Multiple personality: diagnostic considerations. J Clin Psychiatry 41:330-336, 1980

14. Coons PM: The differential diagnosis of multiple personality. Psychiatr Clin North Am 7:51-67, 1984

15. Greaves GB: Multiple personality: 165 years after Mary Reynolds. J Nerv Ment Dis 168:577-596, 1980

16. Kluft RP: Introduction to multiple personality disorder. Psychiatric Annals 14:19-24, 1984

17. Putnam FW, Post RM, Guroff JJ, et al: 100 cases of multiple

personality disorder. Presented at the Annual Meeting of the American Psychiatric Association as New Research Abstract #77, New York, 1983

18. Elliott D: State intervention and childhood multiple personality disorder. Journal of Psychiatry and Law 10:441-456, 1982

19. Fagan J, McMahon PP: Incipient multiple personality in children: four cases. J Nerv Ment Dis 172:26-36, 1984

20. Weiss M, Sutton PJ, Utecht AJ: Multiple personality in a ten-year-old girl. Presented at the American Academy of Child Psychiatry, Washington, DC, 1982

21. Kluft RP: Hypnotherapy of childhood multiple personality disorder. Am J Clin Hypn (in press)

22. Sizemore CC, Pitillo D: I'm Eve. Garden City, New York, Doubleday, 1977

23. Stoller RJ: Splitting: A Case of Female Masculinity. New York, Quadrangle, 1973

24. Goodwin J, Owen J: Incest from infancy to adulthood: a developmental approach to victims and their families, in Sexual Abuse: Incest Victims and their Families. Edited by Goodwin J. Boston, John Wright/PSG, 1982

25. Levinson J, Berry SL: Family intervention in a case of multiple personality. Journal of Marital and Family Therapy 9:73-81, 1983

26. Brown GW: Multiple personality disorder, a perpetrator of child abuse. Child Abuse Negl 7:123-126, 1983

Childhood Multiple Personality Disorder: Predictors, Clinical Findings, and Treatment Results

Richard P. Kluft, M.D., Ph.D.

8

Childhood Multiple Personality Disorder: Predictors, Clinical Findings, and Treatment Results

The development of multiple personality disorder is thought to begin during childhood. It is generally assumed that those individuals who are found, as adults, to suffer multiple personality disorder had initiated and perpetuated the use of dissociative defenses in an attempt to adapt to and survive overwhelming early experiences and their sequelae. The likelihood of childhood onset enjoys such widespread consensual acceptance that it has been incorporated into the Diagnostic and Statistical Manual of Mental Disorders, Third Edition (DSM-III): "Onset of Multiple Personality may be in early childhood or later" (1, p. 258). However, an examination of the literature prior to 1982 reveals little beyond clinical anecdotes to document or corroborate this assumption. The degree of agreement has been more substantial than the evidence marshalled to support it.

Most data cited to describe the existence and manifestations of multiple personality disorder in childhood are drawn either from reports offered by patients in therapy, or from autobiographical and biographical accounts in books written for general audiences (2-7). These descriptions can be impressive and convincing within the contexts of their own narrative processes. However, as potential sources of scientific data, they must be scrutinized with a keen appreciation that memory is an active process, not a passive and pristine recording of historical events. Retrospective recollection is prone to several forms of distortion, revision, and reworking. Furthermore (and without implying disregard for or disbelief in patients' representations), unless there is documentation from sources other than the person who is recounting his or her life, it is difficult to transpose what is offered, however convincingly, from the realm of retrospective account into the domain of scientific record.

Under clinical conditions, such a standard of "proof" is not pursued routinely. Nor, in most circumstances, would it be appropriate. The business of psychotherapy is the healing of distressed individuals. The therapist who forfeits the role of healer and assumes the stance of detective is likely to compromise his or her treatment efforts. It is a therapeutic commonplace to find psychological reality accorded to events and circumstances that can neither be proven nor disproven, and may well be admixtures of fantasy and reality.

With regard to lay accounts, material may have been selected with primary attention to literary representation and expository dramatization, and not to scientific objectivity. Some censorship may have been exerted to protect significant others or one's own amour propre. In exploring new and potentially controversial areas, it is preferable to have second-hand or retrospective data substantiated by the data of actual observation before they are regarded as established. Such information is a sounder source of hypotheses to be explored than a source of firm conclusions.

These cautions are intended neither to discount nor to devalue the contributions of those who have attested to the dangers of assuming that a patient's accounts of traumatization are fantasies rather than realities. It is regrettable that the healing professions have been loath to accept patients' accounts of repugnant and bizarre experiences as data that may reveal actual experiences. Unpleasant truths may be dismissed as distortions or confabulations. Recently, a number of authors have addressed this problem, some speaking primarily as critics of psychoanalytic theory (8), and others as clinical investigators exploring the realities behind the accounts offered by patients (9; Chapter 1 of this monograph).

The issue of documentation becomes especially important in the study of multiple personality disorder. Skepticism and misgivings about the existence, prevalence phenomena, and etiology of the condition have contributed to its being under-studied and under-diagnosed. The increasing recognition, diagnosis, and treatment of multiple personality disorder creates a new urgency in resolving many questions that have long remained unsettled. It becomes critical to study the natural history of multiple personality disorder. To cite two diametrically opposed hypothetical possibilities: On the one hand, if no childhood multiple personality disorder or antecedents to multiple personality disorder could be documented, it would suggest that the condition indeed may be largely factitious or artifactual. On the other hand, if multiple personality disorder (a disorder of considerable morbidity, already shown to be more common than generally recognized) also can be demonstrated to begin in childhood, it would suggest that massive efforts should be undertaken to identify childhood cases and initiate their treatment.

This chapter will describe the evolution of a screening instrument for the early identification of potential childhood multiple personality disorder cases. It will describe the identification of five such cases between 1978 and 1983, will present these cases, and will detail their responses to treatment.

REVIEW OF THE LITERATURE

The literature regarding multiple personality disorder in childhood is rather sparse. My own review indicates that both child psychiatry and the study of child abuse have virtually neglected the subject. Fagan and McMahon (10) came to similar conclusions. Philip Coons, M.D., coauthor of an extensive bibliography of articles pertinent to multiple personality disorder (11), kindly reviewed his voluminous materials to confirm these findings.

The first published account of multiple personality disorder in childhood was Despine's report of his patient "Estelle," printed in 1840 (12). Despine was treating an 11-year-old girl who appeared to be paralyzed. He learned that she hallucinated being comforted by angels, and began to consider a "magnetic" (that is, hypnotic) condition. When he interviewed the patient under hypnosis, he encountered a helper personality, a "guardian angel." Soon, Despine found another personality that lacked paralytic symptoms. In the course of approximately six months of treatment, Estelle became able to walk in her presenting personality, and the personalities integrated. Ellenberger's follow-up data indicates she appeared to have retained her gains (12). In my review of Despine's treatment methods and his stance toward his patient (13), I observed that this pioneer, working alone in 1836, had discovered many of the principles underlying the hypnotherapeutic approaches to multiple personality disorder that had begun to reappear in the literature of the 1970s and 1980s (14, 15).

Although it is known that Wilbur had identified multiple personality disorder in a 12-year-old girl, a fact mentioned in the "Epilogue" of *Sybil* (5), the first contemporary report of a childhood case was made when I presented data on the diagnosis and successful treatment of multiple personality disorder in an eight-year-old boy to the 1979 American Psychiatric Association course, "Multiple Personality: Finding and Fusing," directed by Ralph Allison, M.D. (16). I made additional presentations in subsequent courses, describing two cases in 1981, three cases in 1982, and five cases in 1983. The treatment of the first child (called "Tom" in this chapter) was noted incidentally in a 1982 article (14). Weiss et al. described the occurrence of multiple personality disorder in a 10-year-old girl at a meeting of the American Academy of Child Psychiatry in 1982 (17). In 1984, Fagan and McMahon described the syndrome of incipient multiple personality disorder in four children (10), and I described five childhood cases of multiple personality disorder (13).

The first of the above papers (16) is extremely valuable. It forges a link between relatively unstructured early dissociative phenomena and multiple personality disorder. However, only one case example in that paper, number 2 (Susan), is both a child and shows signs that clearly define the presence of multiple personality disorder. Case examples 1 and 3 show less structured dissociative phenomena. The clinical materials suggest that, failing therapeutic interventions, these cases might have gone on to develop full-fledged multiple personality disorder. Case example 4 illustrates multiple personality disorder in an adolescent girl of 14. This paper offers useful suggestions for screening for childhood multiple personality disorder.

My paper (13) describes five children (aged eight, eight, nine, nine, and 11 at time of diagnosis) in whom other personalities were clearly documented, and mentions two cases known to Braun (ages three and eight). It describes a 16-item atheoretical predictor list generated in 1978. Both papers (10, 13) cite a predictor list derived by Putnam (19). Two additional papers describe hypnotherapeutic (20) and family psychiatric interventions (21) that have proven useful with such patients.

These studies indicate that childhood multiple personality disorder can be identified and treated rapidly and successfully. Fagan and McMahon found that family interventions and play therapy proved effective (10); I discovered that family interventions and hypnotherapy yielded good results (13, 16, 20, 21). In addition, I have offered follow-ups on some of my cases, indicating that the potential for stability is good if retraumatization can be avoided, and that retraumatization can result in relapse.

THE ABSENCE OF CHILDHOOD MULTIPLE PERSONALITY DISORDER FROM PSYCHIATRY

My early experiences with multiple personality disorder suggested but did not prove that the disorder existed in childhood. I learned that its treatment in adults can be arduous and prolonged. I spent considerable time and effort attempting to find common psycho-dynamics among multiple personality disorder patients in order to explain the condition's genetics, and exploring their transference paradigms to discern developmental commonalities. In brief, the patients proved remarkably diverse; what held true for one or some could not be generalized. These researches, reported elsewhere (22), did not allow me to infer how multiple personality disorder might appear in youngsters.

Another avenue of study proved more productive. I reviewed

Table 1. Factors Relevant to the Non-Recognition of MPD in Childhood

1. No index of suspicion by treating professionals or concerned others.
2. Presenting symptoms in one particular personality suggested another more commonplace and familiar condition.
3. Fluctuating findings suggested borderline, psychotic, ictal, or learning disability diagnoses.
4. Ready availability of more familiar explanations for specific manifestations of dissociative behaviors (lying, imaginative play, seizure disorder, imaginary companionship, primitive and/or shaky ego functions, failures of cohesion of self and/or object representations).
5. Children's being unaware of their circumstances and/or condition.
6. Children's withholding data:
   a) They were disbelieved or punished for efforts to communicate their plight.
   b) They suppressed personalities and evidences of them for fear of consequences.
   c) They restricted personalities' manifestations to solitary moments.
   d) There was collusion of personalities to pass as one.
7. The form differs from the adult condition:
   a) An inner sense of separateness may antecede overt expression (some but not all cases).
   b) In some cases there may be a gradual evolution toward the adult form.
   c) An attenuation of outward expressions of differences may exist due to the child's fewer resources and limited degrees of freedom.
   d) Children more readily suppress manifestations of alters due to fear of consequences from adults.
   e) There is closer proximity of childhood MPD structures to the developmental substrates upon which they are built.

the records of 20 successfully treated adult cases in order to learn how these patients might have appeared as children, and to gain insights as to why their multiple personality disorder had not been recognized early in life. These patients satisfied stringent fusion criteria (14, 23) and their stabilization involved no medication. All had been diagnosed without the use of hypnosis. Entries relevant to patients' manifesting and experiencing (or not manifesting and experiencing) evidences of dividedness as youngsters were extracted from their charts, recollections, and from reports from persons, authorities, and agencies having had contact with them during childhood. The patients themselves were asked to reflect on why their situation had not been appreciated. It was understood that ancillary data sources were likely to be prone to several types of systematic bias, among which were denial on the one hand, and retrospective reinterpretation of events by those who now knew that the patient was alleged to have multiple personality disorder, on the other. Factors considered relevant to nonrecognition are listed in Table 1.

Most of the factors in Table 1 are easily understood. No patient's materials included mention of the possibility of multiple personality disorder. Most professionals and agencies queried were either unfamiliar with or were skeptical about the condition. Consequently, the diagnosis of multiple personality disorder had never been considered during these patients' childhoods. Invariably, the patient's symptoms in a major personality had suggested a more well-known and conventional diagnosis to professional informants. Lay sources often relied on rather judgmental, "common-sense" descriptions of the child's symptoms: "liar," "bad," "absent-minded," "possessed," and so forth. When several personalities had been active over a period of time, their kaleidescopic and fluctuating presentations were often understood as signs of severe ego weakness, petit mal and/or psychomotor epilepsy, or of some learning disorder with or without a hyperkinetic component.

It is hard to conceive of a single manifestation of multiple personality disorder which, in isolation, could not be explained by some much more familiar mechanism. The patients' materials were replete with detailed descriptions of classic dissociative phenomena, understood and organized within different conceptual frameworks. For example, one man's alters' amnesias, different voices, and divergent behaviors were understood as the expression of imaginative play, which he stubbornly refused to abandon despite the passage of years.

Most histories and clinical notes indicated that the personalities predominating during childhood did not fully understand the nature of their circumstances. In some cases, they simply were unaware that anything abnormal was going on. Others did not realize that their discontinuous experiencing of time was unusual. For them, it was all they knew, and they assumed that it was normal. Many who heard voices assumed everyone had inner voices. Most accepted the consequences of their disorder as in some way related to their being "bad," and accepted the perjorative interpretations of their behaviors given by those in their environments. Analogies between such a stance and that of the depleted host personality in a classic adult case are readily apparent.

The issues raised by factors 6 and 7 in Table 1 may require further discussion. Many patients recalled their efforts to hold back evidences of their situations. Most had tried to tell some adult of their situations. In the vast majority of cases, they were disbelieved, not taken seriously, or punished. Sometimes a teacher, school counselor, youth group leader, or doctor tried to intervene, but, inevitably, this intervention led nowhere. When personalities became aware of other personalities and learned that the others' emergence or actions caused difficulties, they tried to suppress the others. A common sequence was: 1) the development of an alter with reactive anger and aggression against abusers; followed by 2) its emergence against the abusers; followed by 3) extreme retaliatory aggression by the abusers; eventuating in 4) other alters' suppressing the angry alter for fear of enduring even greater abuse. Many patients' personalities reported that when they were young, their emergence was restricted to solitary moments, often in the privacy of their bedrooms or special hiding places. They sometimes said this was because of "problems" when the alternate personalities emerged with other people around; they often added that this pattern allowed them to be concealed safely not only from others, but also from the host personality, who would get no feedback about their existence or behaviors. A number of patients had simply realized across personalities that it was more expedient to pass as one, and did so from early in childhood.

The patients' accounts also suggested that certain differences existed between adult and childhood manifestations. Many patients had personalities that reported they were separate for years before they "came out" and assumed executive control. Often these alters had talked inwardly to other personalities, but had not asserted behavioral dominance. Several patients reported having had early unstructured "personalities," some of which subsided, and others of which became more elaborate and overtly different over time. The early personalities were vehicles or containers for experiences that the patient disavowed or repressed, and had little narcissistic investment in separateness or distinctness per se. There are some analogies between these observations and those offered by Braun and Sachs (see Chapter 3 of this monograph). However, some patients' histories suggested that marked distinctness was present from the first. In such cases, identification or introjection played major roles in the structuring of personalities.

It may seem obvious, but the child has fewer opportunities or resources to invest in separateness. Hence, it stands to reason that the child's personalities' expressions of differentness may be attenuated, since they may not have highly visible vehicles for the overt demonstration of separateness. For example, an adult's alters may have separate wardrobes, distinct food preferences, and different social circles; a child's alters may have favorite T-shirts, preferred desserts, and may have different preferred friends to play with at recess. An adult's alters might take over and surface in another state, while a child's might prolong the walk home from school. Since the child cannot easily escape those on whom he is dependent, there is great inner pressure to prevent emergence of personalities that would cause difficulties with authority figures. They may not achieve behavioral as opposed to intrapsychic autonomy until adolescence or, in some cases, until the patient leaves the parental home. Lastly, the development of personalities depends upon the availability of substrates that have their own developmental timetables and processes. Consequently, emergence of personalities might depend upon other maturational and developmental processes.

THE PREDICTOR LIST

With these considerations in mind, I generated an atheoretical predictor list for childhood multiple personality disorder, which is reproduced in Table 2. These items were drawn from the records of 20 successfully treated multiple personality disorder patients, as noted above.

The items were designed to tap indices that could be pursued without incurring major denial from a family eager to conceal the abuse of a child from the interviewer, and without incurring the

Table 2. Childhood MPD Predictors[1]

		Data from Five Cases					Cases Positive for Predictor
	Predictor	1	2	3	4	5	
1.	Intermittent depression	+	+	+	+	+	5/5
2.	Autohypnotic/trance-like behaviors	+	+	+	+	+	5/5
3.	Fluctuations in abilities, age-appropriateness, moods	+	+	+	+	+	5/5
4.	Amnesia	+	+	+	+	?	4/4
5.	Hallucinated voices	+	+	+	+	+	5/5
6.	Passive influence experiences, phenomena-suggesting	+	+	+	+	+	5/5
7.	Currently active imaginary companionship	−	−	±	−	−	0/5
8.	Disavowed polarized behavior (aggressive, "too good")	+	+	−	+	+	4/5
9.	Called a liar	+	+	−	+	+	4/5
10.	Disavowed witnessed behavior	+	+	+	+	+	5/5
11.	Muted signs of adult MPD	+	+	+	+	+	5/5
12.	Attenuated expressions of MPD	+	+	+	+	+	5/5
13.	Inconsistent school behavior	+	+	+	+	+	5/5
14.	Refractory to previous therapy	N.A.	N.A.	N.A.	+	+	2/2
15.	Dissociators in family	+	?	+	?	+	3/3
16.	Other DSM-III diagnosis possible	+	+	+	+	+	5/5
	Positive Applicable and Available Indicators	14/15	13/14	12/15	14/15	14/15	

[1] Adapted from Kluft RP: Multiple personality in childhood. Psychiatr Clin North Am 7:121-134, 1984

criticism that the interview protocol itself suggested the phenomena of multiple personality disorder. Items 4, 11, and 12 were routinely pursued after other inquiries had been made. It was anticipated that the presence of several such indicators (eight or more) would suggest the child merited clinical assessment for childhood multiple personality disorder. It was clearly an instrument designed to be used in screening and was never regarded as a diagnostic tool. Nor was any score of predictor factors considered "diagnostic."

Most items can be easily understood. Item 1 used "depression" in a non-technical sense, and did not distinguish it from severe sadness. Item 6, passive influence phenomena, referred to several Schneiderian primary signs (24) often considered indicative of schizophrenia, which I have found to be common in adult multiple personality disorder. They can serve as valuable diagnostic indicators (16, 25). Items 11 and 12 refer to the considerations enumerated in factors 6 and 7 in Table 1. Since 1978, it has become clear that the phraseology of these items is unfortunately vague. By "muted signs" were meant signs of multiple personality disorder that were incompletely expressed because it appeared they were being partially suppressed, "seen through a veil," or appeared to reflect personalities in conflict over dominance. Clinicians without considerable familiarity with multiple personality disorder have found this indicator difficult to use. By "attenuated expressions" were meant signs that might well have been more openly expressed if the child had the opportunity to do so, as in the "T-shirt versus wardrobe" example cited above. I was quite surprised by the failure of predictor 7, which was counter to expectation. I wonder if cases closer to the age at which imaginary companionship is normative might be more likely to be positive for that predictor. In clinical practice, accounts of transitions of imaginary companions into alters are very common.

As Table 2 indicates, these predictors proved quite consistent with the clinical realities of those childhood multiple personality disorder cases that later came to my attention. I used the predictor list in initial interviews with all youngsters in my practice and with other informants. In those patients who proved to have childhood multiple personality disorder, the scores were positive for 90.5 percent (67/74) of the predictors applicable and/or ascertainable in their cases. Nonmultiple personality disorder cases scored 8 or less, but my sample is far too small to serve as the basis for generalizations. It is of note that case example 2, presented below, was referred as a boy with "childhood psychosis." Multiple personality disorder only entered the differential diagnosis on the basis of the predictor score of 12/13. He was about to be hospitalized in a long-term facility because he was dysfunctional at school and at home. Correctly diagnosed and treated, he was retained in school. Within a few months he was unified, behaviorally unremarkable, popular with his peers, and an "A" student.

CASE PRESENTATIONS

Case Example 1 will be described in some detail; the rest will be described quite briefly. Other aspects of these cases are described elsewhere (13, 18, 20, 21). A glossary of terms commonly used in reports on multiple personality disorder patients has been published elsewhere (25).

Case Example 1

Tom was eight years old when referred by his mother, who suffered multiple personality disorder. The mother's mother was later found to have multiple personality disorder. One of the grandmother's alters acknowledged her abuse of the mother. Tom was usually a model child, but he could, abruptly, become exceedingly difficult and disavow having exhibited any good behaviors, even those that had been exhibited just moments before. He appeared to lie flagrantly. He vigorously denied his participation in deeds that his mother, father, brothers, and teachers had witnessed. His voice, speech, body language, and friendship patterns varied with what appeared to be his "moods." At times, he said he was a girl, and behaved effeminately. He admitted, with great embarrassment, that he thought about being a girl. However, he had no recall of ever acting like one. He was accident-prone and seemed unable to learn from experience. His school performance was erratic in the extreme. It often appeared that he had not learned certain subjects; when confronted, he insisted that he had never been taught them. His teachers believed he was slow or learning-disabled. He often said that items of clothing in his closet were not his, and became upset when his mother tried to remind him of shopping trips and their purchasing them together. The boy was frequently depressed, especially after being called a liar or being confronted about disavowed behavior. He was aware of his efforts to cover up memory gaps; he knew he often "spaced out." He acknowledged hearing voices in his head, both male and female. He told me that he had a trick that sometimes helped him remember. When I asked if he would show me this trick, he executed a maneuver known to students of hypnosis as the Spiegel eye-roll (26). It was clear he was using an autohypnotic method of memory retrieval. During the interview, several patterns of different behaviors and voices were noted, and there was ample evidence of intra-interview amnesia.

However, overt separateness was neither inquired after, acknowledged, confronted, nor sought out. Fourteen of 15 applicable predictors were positive.

By the time I assessed Tom, I had undertaken a number of studies to ascertain the safety of the use of hypnosis in treating and assessing multiple personality disorder patients. I decided to explore further using hypnosis, having already made the diagnosis by observation alone. No sooner was eye-closure achieved in the course of an hypnotic induction, than a deep-voiced personality emerged unbidden. He said his name was Marvin, and that he was a spaceman. He advised me of Tom's need for help, "because he wants to be a girl." I asked how he thought treatment could help. He declined to speak, but he wrote advice in a clumsy scribble: "Maybe just ask him if he (Tom) can think of how it was when he was smaller." Tom was amnestic for Marvin's conversation with me. When he wrote the advice message from dictation, his handwriting differed from Marvin's.

This youngster proved to have five alters. Tom was depressed, depleted, and symptomatic; that is, a classic "host" personality. Marvin was a helper in the face of unacceptable anger and fear. Reasonable and resourceful until his coping mechanisms were exhausted, he then behaved aggressively. By the end of therapy, it was clear that Marvin was based on the television program "Star Trek"'s Captain Kirk and television's "The Hulk." At a deeper level, these figures were clearly representations of his father when rational and when brutal. Teddy had a similar role, but, after exhausting rational alternatives of action, reacted by feigning indifference and blocking out feelings. He acknowledged some resemblance to "Star Trek"'s Mr. Spock. However, his behavior pattern clearly paralleled his mother's coping style. The sources of Marvin and Teddy's names remained obscure. The two female personalities, Wilma and Betty, had names that were taken from "The Flintstones," a television cartoon series. Their characteristics were those of mother. It was instructive to note that there was no evidence of borderline types of splitting in the structure of the alters, or in the alters' perceptions of themselves or others.

In terms of the personalities' degree of definition, Marvin achieved DSM-III levels of distinctness. Teddy satisfied criteria A and B, but not C, and the others fused so rapidly that they could not be studied. It appeared that the patient had dissociated in connection with a near-death experience at about the age of 2½. He had fallen into a pond and nearly drowned. He appeared lifeless prior to resuscitation. He had also used dissociative defenses when his father used excessive corporal punishment.

Tom responded rapidly to family interventions and individual hypnotherapy. I have followed him for six years subsequent to fusion, and have screened him for dividedness every one to two months over that period. He has shown no residual tendencies to fall back upon dissociative defenses. He recently suffered a serious accident and coped with it quite successfully. Hypnosis cannot elicit any evidence of separateness.

Case Example 2

This 9-year-old boy was believed to be deteriorating into a childhood psychosis. Referral materials described rapid fluctuations of appearance, attitudes, and competence. His grades were deteriorating, his behavior was becoming bizarre, and he was becoming isolated from his peers. He reported inner voices, amnesias, and poor memory. He said he often was accused of being a liar; he sensed that some other force that he could not control was making him do things against his will. He believed he was possessed or controlled by monsters. Thirteen out of 14 applicable predictors were positive. Once therapy began, he spontaneously dissociated in session. Other personalities emerged. All were named. They differed in voice and behavior, but were not complex. Some expressed unacceptable impulses; one revealed abuse experiences. As has already been noted, he was treated successfully.

Case Example 3

Since 1974, I have routinely met and usually assessed the children of my multiple personality disorder patients, because it seemed plausible that either parental neglect or abuse, family chaos, or identification with multiple personality disorder parents might predispose such children to the development of multiple personality disorder. Therefore, I had assessed this particular boy, the son of a multiple personality disorder mother, just before his sixth birthday. At that point, I found no evidence of multiple personality disorder or dissociative defenses, but noted a strong Spiegel eye-roll (26), suggestive of dissociative potential.

When the boy was eight years of age, he was referred for suspected multiple personality disorder by a protector personality of his multiple personality disorder mother, who stated that "she" (that is, the mother in another personality) had abused him badly. In his initial interview, I learned that he had auditory hallucinations, amnesias, rapid fluctuations of appearance and voice, deteriorating school performance, and a separate unnamed "scared" personality. Twelve out of 15 indicators were positive.

I observed mother and son together. Whenever mother switched into an angry alter, the son switched into the "scared" alter. The boy's most prevalent personality denied being abused and could not believe his mother would beat him. Six months after a successful treatment his mother abused him again. I found he now had developed a very elaborate aggressive personality, identifying with the mother's most aggressive personality. This personality was much more invested in separateness, and required more treatment than had the first. This youngster has sustained unification for over two years.

Case Example 4

This 12-year-old boy was hospitalized while still 11 years of age. He had threatened to kill his adoptive family. He was noted to be amnestic for episodes of intense emotional expression. At such times, he seemed different in voice, accent, and demeanor. His attending physician tentatively diagnosed multiple personality disorder. During my consultive assessment, shortly after his twelfth birthday, he acknowledged an inner accented voice that urged aggressive acts. A corresponding alter was found. It saw itself as dedicated to reunion with the biological mother. Evidence suggested two other alters.

Case Example 5

This 9-year-old boy was suicidal. He had a history of chaotic and disruptive behavior. Clinicians had noted frequent behaviors suggesting a trance-like state. Two styles of behavior were noted. In the first, he was depressed, lethargic, and often dazed; in the second, he was aggressive, vigorous, alert, and always in trouble. In the first, he was partially amnestic for his behavior in the second; but in the second, he recalled all actions of the first. Each was different in voice, speech patterns, and movement characteristics. The first bore his current legal name. The second bore the name with which he was born—his father's name. The boy was three years old when his father died.

Table 3.   Degrees of Personality Definitions

Case Number	Number of Personalities (Including Host)	A Formes Frustes Minimal Definition	B Attenuated	C Transitional or Evolving Toward Adult Form	D Adult Form
		Personalities Best Described as			
1	5		2	1	2
2	6	4	1		1
3	3			1	2
4	4	2 classification uncertain, but A or B			2
5	2				
Totals	20	6	3	2	9

Shortly thereafter, his mother had changed his name. This youngster achieved unification, but no follow-up was possible.

The presentations of these five patients varied considerably in their resemblances to the adult form of multiple personality disorder. This is reflected in Tables 3 and 4. The observations here suggest the childhood case is likely to be less complex than the adult case, and that in some cases, vaguely formed personalities play major roles in the complement of alters. Subtracting the host or presenting personality from those which are in the adult form classification, four cases would satisfy current DSM-III criteria (that is, have at least two alters of a classic degree of complexity), if those criteria are understood in the context of a child's life space. The fifth case was marginal.

The personality types encountered are classified in Table 5. In contrast to adult forms, persecutor personalities, common in adult cases, are notable for their absence here. Also missing are pure inner self helpers (ISH's) as described by Allison (27). It is of note that no persecutors of pure ISH's were described in Fagan and McMahon's child cases (10). My case material suggests that ISH's develop from further specialization of early helpers. This case material also suggests that persecutors develop from the masochistic turning inward of expressions of hostile affect, and from

Table 4. Comparisons Between Adult and Childhood MPD

		Adult	Child
1.	Presence of two or more personalities	Pathognomonic	Pathognomonic
2.	The dominant personality determines behavior	Generally true, but covert influences of nondominant ones are frequent	Usually true, but others commonly try to exert influences without overt emergence
3.	Each personality is complex and integrated with its own unique behavioral and social patterns	Usually in at least some personalities	Expressions of difference may be muted and attenuated
4.	Number of personalities	Two to over 100	Two to six reported
5.	Personalities have strong narcissistic investments in retaining separateness	Common	Not reported
6.	Personalities consciously elaborate and emphasize their differences	Common and often strong	Not reported
7.	Personalities resistant/ apprehensive re: fusion	Common	Uncommon
8.	Persecutor personalities	Common	Not reported
9.	Inner Self-Helper personalities	Frequent	Not reported
10.	Special purpose fragments	Common	Not reported
11.	Systems of personalities	Not infrequent	Not reported
12.	Special personalities or coalitions which handle school or work	Common and often successful	Infrequent and often unsuccessful
13.	Time loss or distortion	Yes	Yes
14.	Skill in covering up time loss	Varies but usually good	Varies but usually poor
15.	"Depression" in host	Common and persistent	Common but transient
16.	Somatoform complaints	Common and pronounced	Uncommon and vague
17.	Severe headaches	Common	Not reported
18.	Use of "We"	Occasional	Rare
19.	Hallucinated voices	Common but usually denied	Very common and usually admitted
20.	"Fugue" episodes	Brief to prolonged, often very obvious because of travel	Brief and often unrecognized
21.	Therapy	Difficult and often prolonged and stormy	Apparently not difficult, usually brief, and marked by steady improvement

Table 4. Comparisons Between Adult and Childhood MPD—Continued

	Adult	Child
22. Useful Techniques	Specialized techniques often essential	General therapy skills and minimal special techniques effective
23. Importance of environmental interventions in therapy	Variable	Essential
24. Relapses	Common and related to other alters, or incomplete abreaction, working-through or memory retrieval	Uncommon. Only reported instance was related to retraumatization

Table 5. Personality Types Encountered

Case Number	Number of Alters	"Typical Host"	Protector of Other Alters	Expresses Forbidden Impulses	Scared, Recalls Traumas	Other
1	5	1	2	2		
2	6	1		2	3	
3	3	1			1	1 Identification with traumatizer
4	4	1		1	1	1 Protector of biological mother
5	2	1			1	Preserving memory of and identifying with deceased father
Totals	20	5	2	5	5	3

helpers who come to feel that they are taking all the suffering for the others; and, as they come to resent it, these persecutors identify with the aggressor's stance. This formulation is untested and quite tentative. Case 3, a week after retraumatization, had an alter who was identifying with the aggressor and was scornful of the host. Perhaps it would have evolved into a persecutor over time.

Table 6 contains the patients' freely offered explanations of their initial and subsequent dividedness, followed by the stated triggers for subsequent divisions, when known. The child who becomes multiple clearly is overwhelmed by traumatic events or

Table 6. Ascribed Etiology of Initial and Subsequent Splits

Case Number	First Split	Subsequent Splits
1	Near death by drowning: age 2½	Excessive corporal punishment; strong unacceptable impulses
2	Autohypnotic efforts to block out family chaos: ages 4-6	Excessive corporal punishment; strong unacceptable impulses
3	Beating by mother: age 7	Beating by mother
4	First separation from biological mother: age 3	Abuse by biological mother: subsequent separations from her
5	Death of biological father and abrupt change of given name: age 3	N/A

circumstances. All five patients had experienced excessive corporal punishment, but only one cited beating as the cause of an initial dividedness. Object loss, separation, physical trauma unrelated to abuse, and the early enlistment of autohypnotic defenses were cited in these other four cases.

It seems reasonable to infer that dissociative defenses are widely used by youngsters who have dissociative potential, both in the face of overwhelming stressors and in augmentation and support of relatively immature nondissociative defenses and coping mechanisms. However, for most youngsters, the adoption of dissociative defenses as an important or predominant mode of functioning may well require the fixing and reinforcing impacts of ongoing exposures to overwhelming circumstances that reinforce the adaptiveness of such extreme measures.

These observations are strongly supportive of the four factor theory of etiology of multiple personality disorder, which I have advanced elsewhere (23, 28). In brief, this theory holds that the child who will develop multiple personality disorder has the capacity to dissociate (factor 1), which is enlisted in defending that child against any of a variety of overwhelming experiences, usually (but not invariably) involving abuse (factor 2). Any of a number of naturally occurring substrates are enlisted to provide the structure of an alter or alters, leading to the remarkable diversity encountered among multiple personality disorder patients (factor 3). The failure of significant others to help the child process his experiences and prevent retraumatization (factor 4) results in a transient pathological adaptation's becoming relatively fixed and further elaborated.

THE TREATMENT OF MULTIPLE PERSONALITY DISORDER IN CHILDREN

The treatment of multiple personality disorder in the adult patient is fraught with difficulty. Although the prognosis is excellent (23), the actual course of the therapy is often prolonged, arduous, and punctuated with crises (28). Its goals involve the alleviation of problematic symptoms and character traits, and achievement of a cooperation among the personalities toward a stable arrangement. This may involve the concession of predominance to one personality, the collaborative cooperation of some or all personalities, or their unification. The latter is both the ideal and the most common outcome, but it may be difficult to achieve in patients who are reluctant to work through traumatic events or whose personalities are deeply and narcissistically invested in separateness. In the treatment of a child, however, his or her restoration to full potential for normal growth and development requires unification.

Despine treated Estelle with hypnotherapy (12). The personalities were allowed and, when necessary, encouraged, to come forth and express themselves. Despine accepted and interacted with all personalities, and treated them with respect. Over a period of time, they unified, and symptomatic behavior was alleviated.

I participated in the treatment of four of the youngsters described above in the case examples. One patient (Case 4) was assessed only. In Case 5, I was one of a team and only made a single intervention. The other three, I treated alone. I used hypnotherapy in three of the four cases I treated (20), and placed great importance on family interventions and agency involvement, both to prevent further traumatization of the child and to alter pathological patterns (21). My work with the families was structured, directive, and undertaken with the families' knowledge that I would not hesitate to invoke legal sanctions to protect the children. I relied heavily upon making and maintaining contact with the personalities, working evenly and openly with all of them, and making sure that each had a chance to express itself fully.

As I have described elsewhere (13, 14, 18, 20–23, 28), this approach does not reinforce dividedness. Instead, by encouraging the alters to identify and empathize with one another, and by offering them a shared experience with the therapist, the dissociative boundaries are eroded. With regard to children, the four factor theory would predict that such a stance would undercut the condition's tendency to become fixed. It has been my experience with these patients and a number of others probably better described by Fagan and McMahon's (10) term "incipient multiple personality disorder," that because 1) children's alters were less invested in separateness; 2) childhood cases did not have inner persecutors; and 3) all proved very motivated for help, the negative therapeutic reactions and crises commonly encountered in adults' treatments did not occur (13, 28). I repeatedly found that the hypnotic interventions useful in adults were effective in children, but often proved unnecessary. Treatments ranged from one to twelve sessions to achieve unification. Additional therapy for other problem areas was more extensive.

Fagan and McMahon (10) relied on play therapy for those among their cases who were between four and eight years of age. They did not specify the format of their unsuccessful treatment of a 14-year-old. It is of note that this latter case behaved like many adults and late adolescents in therapy. Crises were common and resistance was problematic. Their cases of incipient multiple personality disorder appeared to resolve after a minimal number of abreactive play therapy sessions; their case that would qualify for the diagnosis of childhood multiple personality disorder resolved in somewhat over two months of biweekly play therapy.

These treatments had in common the bringing to the surface of repressed issues and the willingness of the therapists to work with the personalities. There was no evidence of attempts to challenge the personalities' existence or separateness, nor were there efforts to suppress them. They were treated with empathy and respect. There was frequent use of imagery techniques to facilitate fusion when this did not occur spontaneously in the course of therapy. Despine and I used hypnotically facilitated imagery. Despine permissively adapted the patient's own images, but I used images tailored to the patients' preferences and dynamics. McMahon used imaginative imagery with "Susan" without specifying whether hypnosis was used, or whether the patient seemed to manifest spontaneous trance phenomena. In sum, the patients who were 11 or younger rapidly achieved the appearance of integration.

There did not seem to be any need to engage in the complex and intricate strategies that often appear essential to treat the adult with multiple personality disorder. Given a supportive therapeutic structure and protection from retraumatization, the patients virtually leaped into health. Follow-up data cited by Ellenberger (12), Fagan and McMahon (10), and Kluft (13) indicate that stable results can be achieved. As noted, I have followed "Tom" for over six years without witnessing relapse behaviors.

The Case of Bobby

It is my policy to interview or at least meet all of the children of my multiple personality disorder patients because it is all too clear that the tragedy of child abuse is often passed from generation to generation. The abusive parent of someone with multiple personality disorder may have been abused, and the patient with multiple personality disorder may have personalities that are abusive to their own progeny. Also, I am concerned about the development of identity in children who identify with multiple personality disorder parents.

Therefore, when Bobby's hospitalized mother was transferred to my care for the therapy of her multiple personality disorder, I assessed her three children. Bobby, Case 3 above, was just under six years old. He had a sister of three and a brother of two. All expressed age-appropriate concerns about their mother's being in the hospital, but showed no dissociative or other major symptomatology. Bobby had a strong eye-roll. They related well to me, to both parents, and to the paternal grandparents. Bobby was very protective of his younger siblings, and showed an evident positive identification with his father. He asked me to make sure his mother came home "real soon."

Bobby's mother proved a complex, resistant, and alloplastic patient. Her course has been stormy in the extreme. Two years later, it was clear that she was one of the most complex cases of multiple personality disorder ever encountered, but that her system of personalities was still largely unknown. During one session, a protector personality took over and expressed concern over Bobby. She said that Bobby was hearing voices, experiencing amnesia, and was frequently showing a separate "scared" personality. She admitted that another of mother's personalities had beaten Bobby several times. That personality was elicited. She admitted beating Bobby, and insisted that he deserved it. She described her own abuse at the hands of her own sadistic father, but maintained such punishment was merited. I asked why. I was told, circularly, that she must have been bad or her father would never have beaten her so severely.

The children were reassessed. Bobby now was eight, his sister was six, and his younger brother was four years of age. The younger brother was uncooperative. The sister clearly blocked out mother's aggressive actions and idealized her. She scored high on the HIP, an index of hypnotizability (26), but there was no sign of separateness. Bobby was positive on 12 of 15 applicable predictors. He denied his mother had ever hit him. Characterologically, he made the same appearance he had made at age six, except that whereas before he had been energetic and buoyant, he now had an overall dispirited and limp demeanor. Hypnotic exploration was undertaken. With Bobby asked to imagine himself in a pleasant situation and not respond to questions, inquiries were made about separateness. An unnamed scared younger personality came forward, and put up its hands as to avert a blow. This alter described the beatings in the same way that the mother's helper and abusive personalities had done. It later called itself "Joey."

Family therapy and individual sessions for Bobby were begun, in addition to his mother's treatment. The mother's personalities refused to promise nonviolence. In one family session, the mother abruptly switched into the abusive personality and began to strike Bobby with closed fists. His eyes rolled upward and Joey, the cowering fearful personality, emerged. He fell to the floor, screaming, and tried to avoid mother's blows. The sister took on a dazed, blank look, and the younger brother hid his head under a pillow. When words failed, I pulled mother off Bobby to prevent severe harm. Restrained, mother went limp, and then her usual personality returned. Bobby's eyes rolled up and his usual personality returned. On inquiry, Bobby and his mother were amnestic for the attack, his sister was partially amnestic, and the younger brother refused to answer questions. Clearly, Bobby had evolved an autohypnotic technique analogous to Spiegel's eye roll induction (26).

Child protective services were involved, and mother's therapy focused on solidifying her control of aggressive personalities. Bobby was treated in individual hypnotherapy (14, 20) and integrated uneventfully in about six sessions. Unfortunately, the mother regressed and beat Bobby severely. Consistent with the conditions of her treatment contract against child abuse, and over her vehement protests, she was committed to a locked facility.

I saw Bobby within one week of the beating. Joey, the scared personality, was not evident. Nor could he be elicited with hypnosis. However, Bobby now had a very complex aggressive personality that had the male version of the name of the mother's aggressive personality that beat him. It was a clear-cut "identification with the aggressor." Bobby abused his siblings in this personality until it was integrated two months later. The traumatic episodes were abreacted, and the aggressive alter received ample hearing. Initially, it had thoughts of disciplining the siblings and of punishing Bobby as well. However, it was persuaded to cooperate. Fusion was facilitated with hypnosis. The integrated personality faced its rage at mother, and repeatedly worked through relevant issues. This integration has been stable for 26 months as of this writing. Bobby's mother has managed to call me or her caseworker each time she feels the urge to beat Bobby. She, herself, is beginning to improve.

COMMENTARY

Clearly, a series of boys with multiple personality disorder is unusual in the literature of a condition alleged to be most prevalent among young adult women. It is my impression that case selection and idiosyncratic factors pertained in the collection of this all-male series. In my series, for example, two multiple personality disorder patients (of whose six children, five were male) trusted me sufficiently to confide their sons' problems. I serendipitously stumbled onto a third while field-testing my predictor list. A fourth was uncomfortable with female therapists and opened up to me. In my area, young female abuse victims are usually referred to female therapists; hence, I rarely see such cases. Similarly, I think the same types of influences, operating in a different direction, led to Fagan and McMahon's presenting a series of girls with incipient multiple personality disorder (10). In all likelihood, neither series stands as an accurate reflection of the male:female incidence ratio in childhood multiple personality disorder.

I am concerned that the multiple personality disorder youngsters who have experienced gross sexual abuse, with premature and traumatic introduction to genital, oral, and anal sexual activity and penetration, may differ from these patients in significant ways. Reconstructing from the childhood recollections of patients who were sexually violated, as well as physically and mentally overwhelmed and abused, I would suspect their presentations would have a higher incidence of somatic complaints, gastrointestinal and genitourinary difficulties, regressive behaviors, overt sexualizations, headaches, and self-injurious and suicidal trends than is reflected in this series. Furthermore, it seems possible that they would be less trustful of the therapist than my patients were and might pose more difficult treatment issues. Due to cultural factors inhibiting female expression of aggression, I would not be surprised to find inner persecutors emerging earlier in sexually violated girls who develop multiple personality disorder.

I also consider it possible that in dissociating youngsters whose ages are closer to those at which imaginary companionship is prevalent, there may be phenomena in which one might see a transition from normative imaginary companionship into imaginary companionship as one of the many possible substrates of a future personality. They might present in such a way as to make distinctions difficult or problematic.

I have similar concerns about evaluating patients whose dissociation might be beginning at the same time as the vicissitudes of self and object representation and the separation-individuation process are being negotiated (29). Putnam's anterospective studies of the subsequent development of children with documented abuse histories, alluded to in Chapter 4 of this monograph may, in time, resolve the concerns raised here.

CONCLUSION

Multiple personality disorder exists in childhood. It can be diagnosed by increasing clinicians' awareness of its existence and by then using a predictor instrument to suggest which children deserve detailed assessments for multiple personality disorder. Once discovered, the condition is very responsive to treatment. Successful therapies act to prevent further traumatization and harm, accord respect and empathy to the personalities, encourage full expression and exploration of feelings, facilitate the coalescing of the personalities, and provide adequate long-term follow-up. They do not end treatment at the point of integration. Instead, they work toward stabilizing gains, enhancing nondissociative defenses and coping, and creating conditions under which normal psychological developmental processes can go forward.

References

1. American Psychiatric Association: Diagnostic and Statistical Manual of Mental Disorders (Third Edition). Washington, DC, American Psychiatric Association, 1980

2. Hawksworth H, Schwarz T: The Five of Me. Chicago, Henry Regnery, 1977

3. Keyes D: The Minds of Billy Milligan. New York, Random House, 1981

4. Peters C, Schwarz T: Tell Me Who I am Before I Die. New York, Rawson Associates, 1978

5. Schrieber F: Sybil. Chicago, Henry Regnery, 1983

6. Sizemore C, Pitillo D: I'm Eve! Garden City, New York, Doubleday, 1977

7. Ward W, Farelli L: The Healing of Lia. New York, MacMillan, 1982

8. Masson J: The Assault on the Truth: Freud's Suppression of the Seduction Theory. New York, Farrar, Straus, and Giroux, 1984

9. Goodwin J: Sexual Abuse: Incest Victims and Their Families. Boston, John Wright/PSG Inc., 1982

10. Fagan J, McMahon P: Incipient multiple personality in children: four cases. J Nerv Ment Dis 172:26-36, 1984

11. Boor M, Coons PM: A comprehensive bibliography of literature pertaining to multiple personality. Psychol Rep 53:295-310, 1983

12. Ellenberger HF: The Discovery of the Unconscious. New York, Basic Books, 1970

13. Kluft RP: Multiple personality in childhood. Psychiatr Clin North Am 7:121-134, 1984

14. Kluft RP: Varieties of hypnotic interventions in the treatment of multiple personality. Am J Clin Hypn 24:230-240, 1982

15. Braun BG: Uses of hypnosis with multiple personality. Psychiatric Annals 14:34-40, 1984

16. Kluft RP: The epidemiology of multiple personality. Paper presented at a course, Multiple Personality: Finding and Fusing (R. Allison,

Director), at the Annual Meeting of the American Psychiatric Association, Chicago, May, 1979

17. Weiss M, Sutton P, Utecht A: Multiple personality in a ten-year-old girl. Paper presented at the American Academy of Child Psychiatry, Washington, DC, 1982

18. Kluft RP: Multiple personality in childhood. Paper presented at the Annual Meeting of the American Society of Clinical Hypnosis, Dallas, November 18, 1983

19. Putnam F: Childhood multiple personality disorder proposal. Unpublished data, 1981

20. Kluft RP: Hypnotherapy of childhood multiple personality disorder. Am J Clin Hypn (in press)

21. Kluft RP, Braun BG, Sachs RG: Multiple personality, intrafamilial abuse, and family psychiatry. International Journal of Family Psychiatry (in press)

22. Kluft RP: The psychophysiology of multiple personality disorder: analytic perspectives. Paper presented at the Annual Meeting of the American Psychiatric Association, Los Angeles, May, 1984

23. Kluft RP: Treatment of multiple personality. Psychiatr Clin North Am 7:9-29, 1984

24. Mellor C: First rank symptoms of schizophrenia. Br J Psychiatry 117:15-23, 1970

25. Kluft RP: An introduction to multiple personality disorder. Psychiatric Annals 14:19-24, 1984

26. Spiegel H, Spiegel D: Trance and treatment. New York, Basic Books, 1978

27. Allison R: A new treatment approach for multiple personalities. Am J Clin Hypn 17:15-32, 1974

28. Kluft R: Aspects of the treatment of multiple personality disorder. Psychiatric Annals 14:51-55, 1984

29. Mahler MS, Pine F, Bergman A: The Psychological Birth of the Human Infant. New York, Basic Books, 1975

9

The Natural History of Multiple Personality Disorder

Richard P. Kluft, M.D., Ph.D.

9

The Natural History of Multiple Personality Disorder

This chapter will describe aspects of the natural history of multiple personality disorder in terms of its clinical manifestations, and will discuss the implications of this natural history for the diagnosis of the condition. The dimensions of the construct of multiple personality disorder will be discussed, and a reassessment of widely held expectations and preconceptions about how this entity presents itself in clinical practice will be made. Toward this end I will review materials that have emerged from three perspectives, and try throughout to address the questions: "What is essential to multiple personality disorder?" "What should the clinician think of when he or she hears this entity discussed or considered in a differential diagnosis?"

The three perspectives alluded to above are those of casefinding research, the study of childhood multiple personality disorder, and the examination of clinical presentations of multiple personality disorder according to the age of the patient at the time of diagnosis.

Casefinding materials stemming from research undertaken between 1976 and 1979 offer a first perspective. They have been presented (1, 2) and referred to elsewhere (3). They were not submitted for publication because their findings were divergent from many of the multiple personality disorder descriptors in the (at that time) about-to-be published DSM-III (4). Their presentation was deferred until DSM-III had become familiar to workers in the field. In the interim, similar epidemiological data were reported by Putnam et al. (5), whose study employed DSM-III criteria. The goodness-of-fit of the data from these two studies was outstanding (F. Putnam, personal communication, 1983). Only some of the implications of the casefinding process per se will be presented here.

From the perspective of recent work on childhood multiple personality disorder (6, Chapter 8 of this monograph), it seemed worthwhile to seize upon the differences in presentation between childhood and classic adult cases, and study whether these differences can cast light upon unexplained and controversial aspects of the adult disorder.

Finally, in the course of studying the multiple personality disorder cases I interviewed personally, it became possible to gain a third perspective: What do multiple personality disorder patients look like when they present for help at different ages? Not only had I observed the presentations of patients from the first to eighth decade of life, but I had also collected a series of patients who refused treatment after being diagnosed, only to return from several months to over a decade later. In these "return" cases, I had the opportunity to compare initial to subsequent presentations, and to learn from the impressions of their interim therapists.

GENERAL CONSIDERATIONS

Multiple personality disorder is in the process of achieving long overdue recognition as a legitimate and important clinical syndrome. Despite increased attention to multiple personality disorder and an upsurge in its recognition in the hospital, clinic, and consulting room, the fact remains that most of these patients, when finally diagnosed, are found to have been under observation for prolonged periods of time before their conditions were discovered. Putnam et al. found that their 100 multiple personality disorder cases had averaged 6.8 years between their first mental health assessment and the accurate diagnosis of multiple personality disorder (see Chapter 8 of this monograph). During that interval, they had received, on the average, over three erroneous diagnoses. My casefinding research found a similar average number of misdiagnoses, and identified a cohort of 20 patients who had been in continuous therapy for over a decade without multiple personality disorder's being suspected (2, 3). All 20 went on to integration; only one continues to need treatment of any sort.

The substantial underdiagnosis and misdiagnosis of multiple personality disorder constitutes a considerable public health problem. Although exceptions are encountered, fully developed multiple personality disorder is associated with considerable suffering, morbidity, and, anecdotally, a substantial risk of suicide. Despite its good prognosis (7), the therapy of florid and entrenched multiple personality disorder can be prolonged and arduous. Data from childhood cases (6, 8–10) suggest that the earlier the condition is diagnosed, the more readily and rapidly it responds to treatment. Delay in the diagnosis and treatment of multiple personality disorder imposes burdensome emotional and fiscal costs on both the afflicted individuals and on society.

In considering the misdiagnosis and underdiagnosis of multiple personality disorder, it is useful to begin by examining challenges to the reality of the problem. There is no dearth of voices proclaiming "disbelief" in the condition's existence or challenging the diagnostic acuity of those reporting large series of such patients. Perhaps, many say, a small number of clinicians are overdiagnosing widely, mistaking artifacts generated by their own enthusiasm for genuine clinical phenomena, and creating a false impression of the dimensions of the problem. It would be inappropriate to deny the possibility of some overdiagnosis by persons with special interest in multiple personality disorder, or by those making a constructive effort to consider the diagnosis, but without prior familiarity with either the condition per se or those entities with which it might be confused (11, 12). The issue is further complicated because different clinicians use different criteria or interpret criteria differently. Bliss, for example, has criticized DSM-III criteria as unduly restrictive (13). Kluft (11) has expressed concern that several forms of multiple personality disorder widely accepted in the nineteenth century literature and described by

Ellenberger (14) are hard to accommodate to DSM-III. Braun (see Chapter 6 of this monograph) and Coons (12) use criteria more stringent than DSM-III.

In reviewing such concerns as overdiagnosis, it is constructive to bear in mind that in most large reported series, the authors are not the parties initiating diagnostic consideration of multiple personality disorder or making the diagnosis. Putnam et al. (5) drew their series of 100 cases from over 90 separate sources. My casefinding research subjects were largely diagnosed by me because the research design, long since abandoned, required all suspected cases to be worked up by the same clinician. However, of the subsequent approximately 140 cases I studied, 85 percent were referred with either documented multiple personality disorder or the diagnosis strongly suspected. They came to me from approximately 90 separate referral sources. In personal communications, Drs. Ralph Allison, Bennett Braun, David Caul, Philip Coons, George Greaves, and Cornelia Wilbur have described similar experiences.

In actual practice, then, the initiation of diagnostic suspicion of multiple personality disorder by many of those who have reported a large number of such cases is a relatively uncommon event. Hence, concerns about a small number of individuals over-diagnosing widely prove unfounded. Instead, a small number of workers to whom many multiple personality disorder referrals have been made for treatment, for consultation, or for research purposes, are reporting the pooled experience of many. When I polled the 70 students at a recent workshop in order to assign them to discussion groups by levels of experience, I was stunned to find the students had encountered 267 nonredundant cases (range 0-20; mean 3.8), none of which had been reported in the literature.

It is prudent to ask whether multiple personality disorder runs the risk of becoming a faddish label. Again, it would be inappropriate to deny the possibility of a period of "trendy" overdiagnosis. Any psychiatrist in the field for a decade or more vividly recalls both the constructive impacts and the over-extensions of innumerable ideas and advances in modern psychiatry. The critical issue regarding multiple personality disorder is that a large number of patients regarded as intractable, correctly diagnosed for multiple personality disorder, have become treatable and have recovered. *The Healing of Lia* is a poignant account of the anguish that faces the incorrectly diagnosed multiple personality disorder patient (15).

Fear of iatrogenesis has prevented many clinicians who note subtle signs of multiple personality disorder from exploring further, especially with hypnosis. Some fear they may "create" or "reinforce" the condition. Although this dilemma has been explored (11, 16), and the risk of iatrogenesis in the clinical setting found to be grossly overstated, many clinicians continue to harbor such worries. In forensic circumstances, such considerations have a more compelling valence and extreme caution is warranted. The reader is referred to a special issue of the *International Journal of Clinical and Experimental Hypnosis* (Volume 32, 1984) for cogent discussions of these matters from several divergent points of view.

Another set of factors revelant to diagnostic problems with multiple personality disorder relate to many clinicians' lack of familiarity with the syndrome, considerable widespread skepticism about multiple personality disorder, and an overall low index of suspicion for any but the most florid manifestations of the disorder. These and the above considerations might be viewed as sufficient reasons for the widespread underdiagnosis and misdiagnosis of multiple personality disorder. Although these considerations are of concern, they speak more to controversies over the status of multiple personality disorder in contemporary psychiatry than to the substantive clinical issues that require attention. They have been acknowledged in recognition of an unfortunate atmosphere of polarization that often surrounds the disorder.

It is my experience that although the factors cited above have considerable importance, the most critical contribution to the problem of the misdiagnosis and underdiagnosis has another source: The natural history of the overt presentation of multiple personality disorder is not widely known or understood. Multiple personality disorder rarely presents as florid multiple personality disorder. The modal natural history of the disorder is not what one would infer or deduce from its classical manifestations. Evidence from 210 personally interviewed cases of multiple personality disorder and a larger number of cases presented by consultees but not seen in person, indicates that multiple personality disorder, viewed in terms of its overt manifestations over a longitudinal time axis, is very different in its appearance from what is seen at those moments in which one is allowed a cross-sectional "vertical" view of its inner structure via the outward expression of that structure in several personalities. In other words, in order to move toward resolution of the misdiagnosis and underdiagnosis problem, one must avoid polemics and ask questions whose answers may contribute to such a resolution:

1. What does multiple personality disorder look like when it does not look like multiple personality disorder as one expects to see it?
2. How can one discover the presence of multiple personality disorder in the absence of its classical manifestations?

This chapter addresses the first question. The second question is the subject of another communication (17). In the process of approaching the first question, possible answers to several vexing clinical problems may be suggested. For example, it may be possible to see why many clinicians can state with candor and conviction that they have never seen a case of multiple personality disorder, and are disconcerted to learn that someone else has made the diagnosis in a patient they once treated. Also, it will be shown that once multiple personality disorder is discovered, it is likely to seem more florid, giving rise to the suspicion that a clinician's interventions are creating it.

An additional set of considerations is pertinent before launching into an essentially descriptive set of observations and data. Elsewhere (7) I have tried to show that multiple personality disorder is a final common pathway rather than the invariable expression of particular dynamics; by analogy, it is a phenotype rather than a genotype. In another context, I have shown that study of the dynamics and transference patterns of a large series of multiple personality disorder treatment cases are notably diverse, and have rejected the hypotheses that multiple personality disorder is invariably a borderline, narcissistic, or hysterical disorder in its core structure (18). Horevitz and Braun (19) have reviewed the relation of multiple personality disorder to DSM-III borderline personality disorder and concur.

A number of authors generalizing from a less extensive data base have reached different conclusions (for example, 20, 21). The absence of a dynamic commonality further complicates the clinical identification of multiple personality disorder. Were there characteristic genetics, conflicts, or transference paradigms, these might prove to be useful diagnostic clues in well disguised cases. At this time, it appears that the aggregate of available data supports the view of multiple personality disorder as a form of childhood post-traumatic stress disorder, a position recently explored by D. Spiegel (22). Hence, its dynamics and structures may vary with the nature of the trauma, the age at which it is endured, and the child's level of development, preexisting ego strengths, and defensive constellations.

CASEFINDING STUDIES

My casefinding work was undertaken in 1976 and discontinued, except for work on screening for childhood multiple personality disorder, in 1979. It consisted of a series of studies in which I attempted to follow up clues from the literature and my clinical experience in order to learn more about the epidemiology and clinical presentations of multiple personality disorder, and to evolve appropriate diagnostic approaches.

My first case was encountered serendipitously in the early 1970s. This raised my index of suspicion, and I found four additional cases by 1975. This caused me to wonder if, perhaps, multiple personality disorder was not as rare as it was alleged to be. I undertook a detailed study of these five patients. All five cases had extensive histories in the mental health care delivery system; all had been diagnosed borderline or schizophrenic (some had received both diagnoses from different clinicians); and all but one had been given an affective disorder diagnosis, as well. None had responded well to prior therapy. All were either trying to hide their multiple personality disorder or to deny it. None were exhibitionistic or inclined to flaunt or augment their pathology. All were masochistic. All admitted they had withheld relevant data at the time of their initial assessments, and all had initially denied amnesia or covered over their amnestic periods. Hence, the patients' actual presentations were counterexpectational to the then-stereotypic picture of multiple personality disorder.

Among the sources I studied, I was struck by Ellenberger's (14) superb review of classic cases and their diverse presentations, and Erickson and Kubie's (23) description of their encounter with an unsuspected alter personality in the course of hypnotic explorations. In addition, I observed that multiple personality disorder patients in treatment revealed signs perhaps more relevant to making the clinical diagnosis than any formal criteria then available, or than any expectations stemming from characteristic features, such as amnesia.

Multiple personality disorder patients in treatment often denied their disorder. In the face of powerful evidence and confrontation, they offered convincing alternative rationalizations to explain away signs and symptoms. They often evaded rather than sought out therapeutic assistance. It became clear that personalities often passed for one another, could emerge and recede so rapidly that the only trace they left was a brief fluctuation in facial expression, and did not necessarily emerge completely to make their presence felt. Often several months passed during which personalities did not emerge fully. They influenced one another by hallucinated inner voices, or in some way by imposing themselves upon alters ostensibly in control of the body.

I realized that a patient withholding or unaware of data, or who initially presented in the manner I often saw in sessions with individuals known to be classic multiple personality disorder patients, would never fall under suspicion for multiple personality disorder. This, and the alleged rarity of multiple personality disorder, led me to believe that multiple personality disorder is considered unusual because 1) clinicians expect to see and confirm a steady and public history of certain dramatic phenomena in order to consider the diagnosis and to document it, and 2) the phenomena they expect to see are not displayed in an ongoing and continuous basis by the majority of multiple personality disorder patients, who try to keep their condition concealed.

Only approximately 13, or 6.2 percent, of a series of 210 multiple personality disorder patients have proven to be flamboyant about their pathology, and less than three percent (all but one among the 13) have responded to therapist's inquiries with attention-catching factitious augmentations of their presentation. In other words, of 100 multiple personality disorder patients, for every seven or eight "histrionic" multiple personality disorder patients, there appear to be 92 or 93 who try to hide their problem and live lives of "quiet desperation." If one includes adolescent cases that are "florid" (though not about their multiple personality disorder), 90 percent are still subdued rather than flamboyant in their presentations. In a personal communication, Thomas Gutheil, M.D., has aptly characterized multiple personality disorder as "a pathology of hiddenness."

When it became clear that multiple personality disorder patients with gross amnesia were denying amnesia, a series of questions about several classes of indirect evidence of amnesia were evolved. Inquiries were made about 1) finding unexplained objects among one's possessions or shopping acquisitions, unfamiliar handwriting in one's domicile, and so forth; 2) noting unexplained changes in other's relationships with one, having people one does not know behave as if they know one, being addressed by a name other than one's own; and 3) school or other experiences in which one could not explain a puzzling absence or presence of knowledge, especially the sense, in elementary school, that everyone else in a class appeared to have been taught something one felt one had not been taught. This yielded some answers that led to initiating work-ups for multiple personality disorder. However, I found that some patients who later proved to have multiple personality disorder had inferred the point of such inquiries and given false negative answers.

This led me to consider hypnotic inquiry as a diagnostic technique. Prior to proceeding, I replicated the procedures described in several experiments alleged to describe hypnotically induced multiple personality disorder. Having discovered that the risks of such an artifact have been highly overstated (11), a conclusion reached independently by Braun (16), I began to use cautious hypnotic inquiries. What is relevant here is that of patients later found to have multiple personality disorder, 56 percent did not reveal their multiple personality disorder in an initial hypnotic assessment. A smaller, more recent sample suggests the same is true of amytal interviews. A multiple personality disorder patient motivated to conceal his or her diagnosis may very well succeed in doing so, despite aggressive diagnostic measures.

Certain clinical experiences led to particular studies. For example, one early multiple personality disorder patient reported feeling compelled to cut herself by a powerful personality whose voice, heard inwardly, commanded her to do so day and night. I asked residents to report any patient who presented with a suicide attempt attributed to an inner voice or a passively experienced compulsion. Over three years, seven of the individuals so referred proved to have multiple personality disorder. In another instance, it became clear that many multiple personality disorder patients' somatic difficulties were relived pains from past traumata, and that medical/surgical efforts to bring relief were of no avail. Consequently, I assessed for multiple personality disorder any patient who had failed to respond to adequate medical efforts for any apparently legitimate somatic complaint. A surprising number of cases were found in this manner, especially among those with cephalalgia, seizures, or gastrointestinal complaints (24).

A similar approach was tried in patients refractory to psychotherapy. A subgroup of 20 patients refractory after a minimum of 10 years of psychotherapy was noted earlier. This overall cohort, however, included patients initially perceived as medication-unresponsive schizophrenics and manic depressives.

It is noteworthy that in the course of several years' experience of testing protocols for multiple personality disorder on individuals believed to be nonmultiple personality disorder controls and volunteers, a small number of multiple personality disorder cases were encountered serendipitously. Once discovered, these patients were very open about their prior efforts to conceal their multiple personality disorder. As a rule, they either declined or did very well in treatment. A few of the patients listed in the "refractory to psychotherapy" group were found in this way.

In psychotherapeutic treatment with multiple personality disorder patients, I observed that they often showed microamnestic behaviors and the classic pictures of simple psychogenic amnesias and fugues. Consequently, I explored all patients referred with any history of any type of amnesia. A dozen multiple personality disorder patients were found in this way, 11 of whom at first appeared to have psychogenic amnesia alone. One patient was pursued after showing microamnesic episodes whenever sadness over termination came under discussion.

A major area of inquiry was stimulated by my background reading for a project on schizophrenia (25). I practiced inquiring about the Schneiderian first rank or primary symptoms of schizophrenia on a research cohort of multiple personality disorder patients. I found that virtually all multiple personality disorder patients not denying their diagnosis had experienced some of these symptoms. Lest inferences be drawn from putative multiple personality disorder patients later proven to have been misdiagnosed schizophrenics, a cohort was assembled, including patients who were able to achieve integration as defined by stringent criteria, and sustain integration a minimum of 27 months without the help of a major tranquilizer, antidepressants, or lithium. Patients still using minor tranquilizers were not excluded. The results are shown in Tables 1 and 2.

Only the first rank symptoms noted on their initial evaluations were tabulated. Additional symptoms reported during the course of treatment were not included, for reasons discussed below. As noted, an average of 3.4 symptoms per patient were acknowledged. Subsequent work indicated that this was a highly cooperative cohort, as might be suspected by their excellent outcomes. Many patients are so anxious that they will not admit such experiences during evaluation, but will do so during therapy. During therapy, however, amnestic barriers are being challenged and the pathology is being altered, so that most multiple personality disorder patients show more signs of analogous phenomena. Hence, tabulations after the initial evaluative sessions were disregarded in this study.

Table 1. The Incidence of First-Rank Symptoms of Schizophrenia in the Presentations of 24 MPD Patients Who Achieved and Sustained Integration

Symptom	Number of Patients with Symptom	Percentage of Patients with Symptom
1. Audible thoughts	0	0
2. Voices arguing	9	37.5
3. Voices commenting on one's actions	5	20.8
4. Influences playing on the body	9	37.5
5. Thought withdrawal	8	33.3
6. Thoughts ascribed to others	9	37.5
7. Diffusion or broadcasting of thoughts	0	0
8. Made feelings	19	79.1
9. Made impulses	12	50.0
10. Made volitional acts	10	41.6
11. Delusional perception	0	0

Adapted from Kluft RP: Epidemiology of multiple personality. Paper presented at the Annual Meeting of the American Psychiatric Association, Chicago, May, 1979.

Table 2. Number of First-Rank Symptoms Reported by MPD Patients

Patients (Total 24)	0	3	7	5	3	1	3	1	1
Number of Symptoms	0	1	2	3	4	5	6	7	8

Average Symptoms per Patient = 3.4

Adapted from Kluft RP: Epidemiology of multiple personality. Paper presented at the Annual Meeting of the American Psychiatric Association, Chicago, May, 1979.

The study of these first rank symptoms has been most instructive. First, it offers valuable clues as to how personalities experience their interactions with one another, especially on the part of those alters who are unaware of the nature of their condition, and believe they are "crazy," or "possessed." Second, it makes available a line of inquiry that taps for diagnostic purposes the types of phenomena often only reported by cooperative and trusting patients after therapy gets under way. Third, asking about these phenomena constitutes a nonintrusive screen for patients meriting further consideration for multiple personality disorder. As such, it is useful in forensic and other settings where special considerations make it essential to avoid any possibility of suggesting the diagnosis.

For example, the author was asked to do a forensic assessment on a woman whose remarkable and uncontrolled violence had led the court to consider forbidding her access to her children. She appeared refractory. If there were no prospects of treating her violence, she would lose her family. The patient had been told about multiple personality disorder, and was assured she did not have it. She had been led to understand that if she had it, she was "crazy," and she, in the host personality that did not acknowledge the violence, reached the erroneous conclusion that if she could persuade the examiner that she did not have multiple personality disorder, she would regain her children. Actually, she was considered untreatable and would lose her children unless she were found accessible to help. She denied every classic sign of multiple personality disorder, but admitted to several first rank symptoms. On this basis, I prolonged the assessment and, after three hours, observed a spontaneous personality switch. I met three other personalities, one of which freely admitted the violent acts. The court remanded the patient to appropriate treatment for multiple personality disorder.

Finally, the casefinding observations (all done prior to DSM-III) raise some intriguing questions. The criteria for multiple personality disorder (300.14) are as follows (4):

A. The existence within the individual of two or more distinct personalities, each of which is dominant at a particular time.
B. The personality that is dominant at any particular time determines the individual's behavior.
C. Each individual personality is complex and integrated with its own unique behavior patterns and social relationships.

The thrust of the casefinding data is that many patients who fulfill these criteria at certain points in their illnesses do not do so at other points. On these latter occasions, they show signs that differ from and even contradict them. For example: When a host, unaware of amnesia or of other alters, experiencing passive influence, acts in a way that is impelled by another alter, one must wonder "who is dominant," "who" is in control, "who" is determining behavior? At that point, the patient would fulfill neither criteria A nor B, and conceivably would not be suspect for multiple personality disorder.

A review of the literature of dissociation with these criteria in mind strongly suggests that criteria A and B rely on a model of dissociation that has been superceded. Naturalistically occurring multiple personality disorder does not conform itself longitudinally over time to what has been portrayed as its classic picture, a picture that appears to embrace classic dissociation theory. Frischholz approaches the theoretical issues raised by different models of dissociation in Chapter 5 of this monograph.

In this context, it is noteworthy that one aspect of the difficulties in diagnosing multiple personality disorder is that the mental health disciplines have come to expect as normative what in fact is a relatively unusual presentation: florid, overt, and unconcealed multiple personality disorder. The very inconsistencies often used to challenge the diagnosis of multiple personality disorder really are normative. Their misinterpretation is an unfortunate consequence of constructing diagnostic criteria that appear to demand compliance with a model of dissociation that has been exceedingly valuable, but is not without certain shortcomings (see Chapter 5 of this monograph).

CHILDHOOD MULTIPLE PERSONALITY DISORDER

In "Childhood Multiple Personality Disorder" (Chapter 8 of this monograph), I described multiple personality disorder in children and contrasted certain aspects of the adult and childhood forms. The following discussion restricts itself to the implications of those differences for the natural history of multiple personality disorder.

Study of children with multiple personality disorder revealed that their personalities often attempted to influence the behavior of the personality in ostensible control of the body without emerging overtly and seizing control in the purportedly "classical" fashion. Passive influence experiences and partial copresences, described elsewhere in terms of the crises they may pose for the adult patient (26), were commonplace. As noted in the previous section, such phenomena challenge a rigid interpretation of DSM-III's criteria, especially Criterion B. For a variety of reasons, in many cases it proves both prevalent and functional that the personalities exert their influence from "behind the scenes." A youngster encountered recently had a personality that expressed aggression by destroying things in the home. It did so by compelling the body to act while the hapless host found itself in the grips of pressures it could neither accept nor control. Inquiry revealed that when the aggressive alter had taken over completely, the boy, in the usual host, denied the acts he had obviously committed, and received additional punishment for "lying." This "compromise" emerged: The aggressive alter imposed its will as an ego-dystonic "made action" that the host experienced and recalled, but could not prevent. The unfortunate host accepted his family's judgment—that he was a "bad kid" who would wind up in jail before long.

As noted in a previous section, such phenomena are counterexpectational vis-a-vis DSM-III, but well within the purview of current theories of dissociation. An appreciation of dissociation and the models advanced to explain it are essential to a contemporary understanding of many aspects of multiple personality disorder. In major current theories of etiology (7; Chapter 3 of this monograph; 27), the capacity to dissociate is assumed to be a precondition for the condition's development. Elsewhere in this monograph, Braun and Sachs (Chapter 3) and Frischholz (Chapter 5) allude to observations that call for a modification of classical dissociation theory, with which DSM-III Criteria A and B are consistent. Both findings in childhood multiple personality disorder and in casefinding research lead to a realization that legitimate multiple personality disorder cases often fail Criterion B in many, if not most, instances. It is crucial for the diagnostician to bear this in mind. This issue will be addressed from another standpoint in a later section.

In childhood cases, many personalities express their differences in a muted or attenuated fashion. As noted, children have comparatively restricted opportunities and resources to elaborate their alters' differences. Furthermore, they were rarely motivated to do so. The alters had little narcissistic investment in separateness compared to what is common in adult cases, and none seemed impelled to make public expressions of difference or "work" at being different. Consequently, while the childhood cases generated or nearly generated alters of sufficient elaborateness to fulfill DSM-III's Criterion C, often alters with less definition were equally important or even more central and active.

This raises a point that is relevant to the natural history of multiple personality disorder: when critical roles are performed by alters of unquestioned autonomy, but which are uninvested and unmotivated in being conspicuously separate, the major external signs of multiple personality disorder are dramatically diminished. In fact, in many adult multiple personality disorder cases eager to evade detection, a large number of alters pass as one, forfeiting external signs of difference. In such cases, once the patient realizes that someone has made the correct diagnosis, he or she may relax and show more overt differences with that individual. I treated a highly regarded scientist who hid his multiple personality disorder from me for a first therapy of five years, and revealed it only in a slip of the tongue in the second year of a second period of treatment. He had successfully concealed the condition from his colleagues, spouse, and children. His alters only expressed their differences in solitude, with strangers, and in what proved to be a successful therapy.

In sum, it appears that whether a patient with multiple personality disorder will fulfill DSM-III Criterion C is more a function of opportunity and motivation than an index of the central pathology. In childhood cases, just as in naturalistically occurring adult multiple personality disorder, it is counterproductive for a clinician to expect to encounter florid manifestations in order to make the diagnosis. In this context, it is instructive to reflect that the striking neurophysiological differences documented in Braun's cases were manifested in "fragments" as well as in fully defined classic personalities (28).

A review of childhood cases indicates that some of the personality types and configurations frequently found in adults are not found in youngsters. This, combined with the considerations raised above, challenges the investigator to wonder whether expectations of how multiple personality disorder should appear are also unduly influenced by unwarranted assumptions about what types of personalities are usually present. These children had no inner persecutors, classic inner self helpers (ISH's), special purpose fragments, or systems of personalities. The alters who expressed either repressed or forbidden impulses rarely were overt about their differences. An adolescent or adult who perpetuated such an arrangement would rarely resemble classical multiple personality disorder.

Reported children with multiple personality disorder have fewer somatoform complaints and headaches than do adults. However, this may be due to sampling selection (see Chapter 8 of this monograph), the way children's alters interact, or because the pain associated with painful traumata is more experience-proximate and consequently requires more intense and complete repression. The implication for casefinding is that if this juvenile pattern persists in a patient, additional common diagnostic indicators fall away.

Other differences between children and adults include adults' more frequent use of "we" statements and children's lesser guardedness about admitting inner hallucinations. It is my experience that "we" statements are more characteristic of multiple personality disorder patients after diagnosis and socialization to treatment, although some patients with "systems" or "families" of alters speak this way quite openly. It may prove to be an overrated diagnostic indicator. It is my experience that adult multiple personality disorder patients may have started their patient careers by openly discussing their hallucinations, but become guarded after finding that this is followed by their being treated as schizophrenics.

In summary, the observations from cases of childhood multiple personality disorder add their weight to the casefinding materials in suggesting that patients who display overt and florid signs of multiple personality disorder consistently over time are the "tip of the iceberg." They are not necessarily the purest or most typical expression of multiple personality disorder. They may have other forms of character pathology that contribute to the openness with which their multiple personality disorder is seen. To anticipate a later argument, in many cases treatment disturbs the homeostatic arrangements among the alters which keeps the condition fairly well concealed. This contributes to the often-dramatic "opening up" of cases beginning in therapy, and the post hoc propter hoc fallacious inference of iatrogenesis or reinforcement by fascination.

THE APPEARANCE OF MULTIPLE PERSONALITY DISORDER AT DIFFERENT AGES

In the course of interviewing a large number of individuals afflicted with multiple personality disorder, it became clear that the condition's manifestations differed in patients who had been diagnosed at different ages. Although the central features persisted and virtually all cases included in this section's discussion satisfied DSM-III criteria at some time while they were under my observation or that of a colleague, it was not unusual for a patient to spend much of his or her life making a different sort of appearance.

This section will review observations on age-related aspects of presentations, intercurrently describe findings in patients who declined treatment after diagnosis but returned years later, and offer some examples of patients' fluctuating presentations over time. The distribution of ages at diagnosis in the author's series has remained consistent as the series has grown. The majority, 80 percent, are diagnosed between the ages of 20 and 50, with approximately 65 percent found between 20 and 40 years of age. Approximately three percent are under 12, eight percent between 12 and 19. Also, about six percent are between 50 and 59, and three percent are 60 or older. The presentations of childhood multiple personality disorder are described in Chapter 5 of this monograph, and summarized in the previous section.

I interviewed 16 adolescents (ages 12–19) with multiple personality disorder. Twelve were female and four were male. It was interesting to note a marked sex-related difference. All four males had aggressive propensities in at least one alter. One committed arson, one attempted robberies, the third bludgeoned victims with a brick, and the fourth, the youngest, was destructive of property. The first three had been involved with the legal system, the fourth had been disciplined in school. They were referred to the mental health system with putative diagnoses of temporal lobe epilepsy, mania, schizophrenia, and Tourette's syndrome, plus character disorder, respectively. They handled their amnesias in ways that raised suspicion as to their veracity. At times, they denied acts they clearly had done, but at other times, they admitted them with bravado. Sometimes, on inquiry, it was clear that they had no direct recall of the acts they admitted. Before his multiple personality disorder was diagnosed, one of the arsonist's alters told me that he had no recollection of setting the fires, but would rather go to jail than be labelled as "crazy." He studied what he was told of his actions to make his case that he was "bad, but not mad," more convincing. Two rationalized their amnesias and disavowed behaviors as drug-related, but admitted that such episodes had occurred at times when drugs were not used.

The 12 girls were a curious group. Only two lived with intact families on a regular basis, and one of those families was quite chaotic. Multiple personality disorder patients from intact families usually are diagnosed at later ages. I think that this is due to ongoing suppression of alters, alters' passing for one another, and families keeping their teenagers out of the mental health system. Some were runaways from incestuous or abusive families. Many were promiscuous in behavior, but some had only second-hand knowledge of such actions. For two, their pregnancies (the origins of which they could not explain) were their only conscious evidence of sexual activity. Five had been raped as they wandered about in a dissociated state or sought refuge among fringe social elements. Three had heavy involvement with street drugs. One was flagrantly sociopathic. Somatoform complaints were common, for which many had received prescriptions of tranquilizers or analgesics. Suicidal gestures, often with these very medicines, were common. Most of these patients (eight, or 75 percent) dissociated floridly in front of me, but switched personalities rapidly without this being openly admitted. They had been dismissed as impulsive, histrionic, ictal, schizophrenic, borderline, "acting out," or a combination of these. Exploration revealed that many experienced a constant inner bombardment of passive influence experiences among the alters. Such rapid fluctuations often are seen in known multiple personality disorder patients in therapy, but are rarely appreciated as a useful diagnostic sign. Many had learned that no one believed them when they disavowed a disremembered action, so, out of despair and/or expediency, their initial denials usually crumbled into false confessions of being liars.

The other four had less of an "adolescent turmoil flavor." They were, as a group, withdrawn. One immature girl of 15 had the structure and characteristics of childhood multiple personality disorder. She rapidly recovered. Two were showing a more typical adult presentation: a neurasthenic and depleted host predominated, but acknowledged amnesias, headaches, and experiences of being confronted with or regaining awareness amidst out-of-character behaviors. The last was a young woman who gave the appearance of deteriorating into a malignant treatment-refractory schizophrenic process. Screened and correctly diagnosed, she was rapidly discharged and went on to attend and graduate from college. She is well on five-year follow-up.

As a group, these adolescents all earned other diagnoses, and most gave the picture of adolescent turmoil. In this group, multiple personality disorder was made as a superordinate diagnosis (29), and, in retrospect, many aspects of their presentations were belatedly appreciated to be dissociative in nature. The eight girls with florid dissociation were the only group encountered which, as a whole, could be described as histrionic, a term often inappropriately overgeneralized to describe most multiple personality disorder. Twenty-five percent declined treatment. As a rule, when such patients returned for treatment, their presentations were markedly different (as in the case of "Cissy," below).

When the alloplastic adolescents' personalities "slowed down" and entered a dialogue with the interviewer, or when the personalities of the withdrawn ones became accessible, their degree of complexity and extent of development varied quite widely, from the barely elaborated to the exceedingly distinct. All personality types might be encountered, and there were some indications of beginning systems or elaborate social networks among alters.

All patients who were seen as adolescents and refused treatment then, but later returned, were markedly different on reassessment. For all of these adolescents, their histrionic appearance had sub-sided. They presented as depressed masochistic hosts whose alters were more structured in their identities and their attitudes toward one another. It is my impression that naturally occurring adoles-cent multiple personality disorder is usually hard to diagnose. Its most prevalent manifestations in many cases are phenomena usually encountered in adult cases only when treatment is well under way, and invariably the patients appear to have another, more common, diagnosis.

The classic picture of multiple personality disorder in adult life is well known, and indices for its diagnosis have been published (3, 4, 12, 30, 31). It is useful to bear in mind as a baseline that most multiple personality disorder patients come for help in a depressed, masochistic, and anxious host alter that appears to be a rather standard "neurotic type." A review of the initial presentations of the patients reveals that few present in a manner that suggests multiple personality disorder. In my series, five percent presented self-diagnosed. In most cases, this was not believed by the initial clinician.

I had the following unnerving experience. Prior to my first multiple personality disorder case, I did not think the condition existed. I saw a young woman who claimed to have multiple personality disorder, and dismissed her claim. She never men-tioned it again. Seven years later, while doing research in multiple personality disorder, I asked her to be a control subject for a new multiple personality disorder screening protocol, since I believed she was a medication-controlled paranoid schizophrenic. A protec-tor personality rapidly took over, cursed at me for disbelieving the patient in the first place, introduced me to other personalities, resumed control, and chastized me vehemently at great length. Thereafter, she left, never to return.

Approximately 15 percent of adult patients are diagnosed when they dissociate spontaneously during assessment or therapy. Another 40 percent show some subtle form of classic signs that could alert the clinician to multiple personality disorder if he or she has an index of suspicion for the condition, and has seen the subtle signs of switching that one observes during the treatment of such patients. The remaining 40 percent show no classic signs of multiple personality disorder and are diagnosed either serendipitously, when the clinician makes a strong effort to pursue diagnostic clarity, when ancillary information raises the issue, or when personalities suppressed in session try to get the clinician to see what is going on (3). One patient was in treatment for six years with a colleague when this colleague began to get letters from the patient's address, but in different handwritings, telling him his patient was one of several personalities.

In exploring the 80 percent who ultimately are diagnosed as having multiple personality disorder but conceal it well under observation for protracted periods, it becomes possible to list certain common presentations.

It is not uncommon for classic multiple personality disorder to be missed simply because no one thought to consider it, or because the alters passed for one another. A retrospective review of process notes on such patients unexpectedly revealed that many had frequently been amnestic for changes in appointments, misheard vacation announcements, asked the same questions repeatedly, disremembered the content of prior sessions, and in a number of ways had shown what I call evidences of micro-amnestic events. One such case was discovered when the patient insisted she had not been told of my planned absence; and I, who recalled notifying her, asked her to free-associate. Shortly thereafter, another alter emerged and said it had attended the session when the announcement was made.

Not infrequently, the emergence of an alter is a low-incidence event, or the patient has a sequential variety of multiple personality disorder (14). In such cases, one personality may be in control for a long period of time, have a continuous sense of itself for years, and the interviewer may have no hint that he is dealing with multiple personality disorder. The patient who drew this to my attention was an older woman who was terminating a long therapy and wept copiously, but denied weeping. I pursued this and learned that I had spent years working with an alter who had been out continuously for 29 years. The termination triggered a little girl alter who saw, in termination, a repetition of the loss of her beloved father.

The above introduces another major reason for the under-diagnosis of adult multiple personality disorder. For many reasons, one alter may so dominate the patient's public presentation that multiple personality disorder shows minimal visible signs. One may suppress the others knowingly or may do so in trying to achieve what it perceives as self-control in the face of inner pressures or voices. A system of personalities may work through one alter; all may learn to imitate one alter. As time goes on, patients with a "one alter predominant" presentation often show increasing flexibility, range, and resilience in that alter, so that others' need for or pressure toward emergence is diminished. Sometimes this is accompanied by a relative atrophy of the manifest differences among the separate alters.

The most common presentation that lends itself to discrete description is the patient who has failed to improve in a straight-forward way when given competent and adequate treatment for medical or mental health complaints. For reasons yet obscure, multiple personality disorder patients' responses to medication may differ widely among alters (32, 33), and what appears to be a bona fide condition may prove to be an expression of interpersonality conflict or somatic memories of past traumata (24). One patient's apparent epilepsy was refractory. It proved to be an expression of alters contending for control of the body. Untreat-able headaches have often proven due to alters' conflicts. A patient received extensive assessment and numerous therapies for leg pains believed to reflect an obscure collagen disease. It was learned that her parents had routinely left her tied up in contorted positions when they left the house. After the memories had been recovered and abreacted, the symptoms ceased.

These examples also illustrate a quite common presentation in patients who are later found to have multiple personality disorder:

the somatoform. Many multiple personality disorder patients spend years consulting physicians for somatic distresses before they enter the mental health system. Often patients who remained in strictly controlled parental homes during adolescence and who concealed their multiple personality disorder begin to present themselves for medical attention. One woman, an incest victim whose alcoholic parents left her unsupervised, roamed the streets in several flagrant alters throughout her teens, and became addicted. In contrast, another, supervised every moment, had alters who emerged only in her bedroom, except for one who did cheerleading and was co-conscious with the host. She was at her family doctor's almost weekly for some complaint. When the latter patient was diagnosed in her 30s, she had been referred to the author for her somatoform ailments. Physical expression of inner turmoil is common in multiple personality disorder, and often remains a persistent adaptation.

Amnesia without hints of multiple personality disorder was commonly encountered, as were dissociative phenomena that were ostensibly part of other presentations. I encountered six patients who were amnestic after auto accidents, and a lesser number who were amnestic after assaults or deaths in the family, who later proved to have multiple personality disorder. Similarly, I found several patients who proved to have multiple personality disorder whose dissociative manifestations were assumed to be part of other syndromes. The inference to be drawn is that multiple personality disorder should enter the differential diagnosis of any patient whose history includes amnesia, depersonalization, derealization, and the like, even if another diagnosis seems appropriate. Putnam et al. (29) have offered cogent arguments that multiple personality disorder is a superordinate diagnosis that will be missed if one stops assessing a patient when criteria for one condition are satisfied. It is a rare multiple personality disorder patient whose phenomena would not allow another DSM-III diagnosis to be made.

A large number of multiple personality disorder patients present with the appearance of psychotic decompensation in a borderline state, or with signs suggestive of a schizophrenic, schizophreniform, affective, schizoaffective, or paranoid psychosis. There is an unfortunate tendency to assume that severe or bizarre symptoms imply a formal psychotic disorder, a tendency deplored by Spiegel and Spiegel (34), Bliss et al. (35), and Kluft (26). Patients experiencing hallucinations and delusions may well be experiencing alters' intercessions. It is a widespread clinical impression that multiple personality disorder patients' auditory hallucinations are usually, but not invariably, experienced as within the head, except when there is simultaneous visual hallucination of an alter's being separate. Most auditory hallucinations in schizophrenics are experienced as originating outside of the head. I have taken to assessing the Spiegel eye-roll (34) of all my patients. While not a definitive measure, this simple procedure helps identify patients whose psychotic symptoms may be related to a dissociative diathesis. In my experience, the majority of psychotic presentations in individuals with high eye-rolls have a dissociative component, and a certain percentage have multiple personality disorder rather than a traditional psychosis. This is crucial to consider because, over time, multiple personality disorder patients misdiagnosed and treated as schizophrenics come to give histories suggestive of schizophrenia, and may become socialized to act in a certain patient role, or identify or model alters upon other patients' deteriorated behaviors.

Well disguised adult patients often present with nothing more to suggest multiple personality disorder than affirmative answers to inquiry about passive influence or special hallucination experiences, the Schneiderian first rank symptoms. These have been discussed in a previous section. The patient who feels his thoughts and actions are not under his control, who feels driven by impulses he does not experience as emanating from his own psyche, who experiences thoughts he cannot account for, and who helplessly performs complex acts in the face of his conscious indifference or resistance to them, may indeed appear borderline, psychotic, or severely obsessive-compulsive. However, the student of dissociation and hypnosis recognizes these as common phenomena of hypnotic and post-hypnotic suggestion and, as such, possible indicators of a dissociative process at work. Retrospective reviews of charts show that such signs, or the special hallucinations of voices commenting on one's actions or arguing within the head, are often noted long before more definitive signs of multiple personality disorder are observed.

Adult patients, especially males, may present as sociopaths or alcoholics. Only one "sociopathic" male in this series had charges pending at the time of diagnosis. All others had been through the legal system in the past and were now seeking psychotherapy. Some maintained they were innocent of the charges against them; but most, whose amnestic barriers had been breached by data they learned during interrogation or trial, had a vague, derealized, or ego-alien recollection. Some had no conventional memory of the event, but had "flashbacks" or visual hallucinations of the crimes. Some recalled the crimes only in dreams. Their multiple personality disorder was discovered in the course of exploring their past criminal experiences, or, in one case, by exploring an urge to commit an offense. One gifted alcoholism counselor, the late Judy Youngblud, of Lancaster, Pennsylvania, found and referred to me nearly a score of patients with multiple personality disorder by meticulously observing "black-out" behaviors in recovering alcoholics who had been dry for over a year. She suspected that in the past their dissociative behaviors had been covered over by intoxication during periods of active addiction. Using Youngblud's experience as a guide, I found an additional six multiple personality disorder patients among recovering alcoholics.

In summary, only about one in five adult multiple personality disorder patients presents with overt multiple personality disorder by self-disclosure or easily recognized dissociation. It is a rare multiple personality disorder patient whose presentation could not suggest another diagnosis. The clinician must be prepared to include multiple personality disorder in every differential diagnosis, and to be aware that as treatment progresses, the signs alluded to above may be subtle indicators of the presence of multiple personality disorder.

Within the adult age range, it is possible to make some generalizations. Many patients diagnosed in their 20s, regardless of their presentations, seem to show more "open" pathologies than those diagnosed in their 30s, many of whom present as depressed, anxious, controlled, and mildly obsessional. Patients diagnosed in their 40s often were very strong individuals of considerable accomplishment, whose pathology was quite well hidden. Often patients diagnosed near or over the age of 30 were found to have managed with some sort of inner homeostasis until some external event triggered a decompensation. Patients over the age of 40 showed the same tendency, but also seemed to be responding to some inner sense that if they did not seek help soon, any chance of changing their pathological adaptations would be lost.

The later a patient was diagnosed, the more likely it was that one alter, of considerable range and resilience, was "out" the vast majority of the time. Exploration of such patients often disclosed that many personalities had atrophied, gone dormant, or had not taken over for years.

Of the patients seen first between 50 and 59, one had classic florid multiple personality disorder, but the rest showed depression, anxiety, and passive influence experiences. This group showed signs that were a natural progression of those just described as increasing with age: increased tendencies toward one alter dominance, and atrophy, simplification, inactivity, and dormancy of alters. Some had spontaneously fused.

To my knowledge, the diagnosis and treatment of multiple personality disorder in the older patient has never been the subject of a published article. I encountered such a case serendipitously in the mid-1970s. I was asked to do a consultation, and in the process to demonstrate the mental status examination to observing students. The patient was a woman in her early 60s. She arrived promptly. She understood that she was to be seen by me in consultation. She was quite cooperative, but when I addressed her by the name on her chart, she insisted that her name was different. Suspecting a simple error of scheduling or a misfiled chart, I proceeded with the examination. I then called the referring therapist to apologize for what I though might have been a snafu. The therapist came to the interview area to resolve the confusion, and said that I had interviewed the correct patient. A comparison of the patient's mental status as elicited by me with that elicited by the therapist revealed marked differences. When the therapist and I saw the patient together, she gave the name on the chart, and was quite different from and amnestic for her appearance during the consultation. Ancillary data sources revealed both patterns of behavior, amnesias, and severe migraines were well known to family members. Her psychiatric history indicated over 30 years in the mental health delivery system under schizophrenic and depressive diagnoses.

This patient showed that classic florid multiple personality disorder exists in older adults. In the last decade, six additional cases have been encountered. One was discovered in a seizure disorder clinic, when a perceptive colleague discerned that the patient's symptoms suggested alters struggling for control. At times, she showed complete dissociation into classic alters; but most of the time she showed a series of spasmodic physical contortions and disturbances of her sensorium as the alters battled for dominance.

While these two showed the persistence of overt multiple personality disorder into the seventh decade, the other five patients' manifestations were quite disguised. One woman who sought hypnotherapy for obesity dissociated into a child alter while receiving relaxation instructions. It was learned that this alter, which became separate after a childhood molestation, came out at times when the patient was alone, and gorged on sweets, while the presenting alter was at a loss to explain her weight gain while on what she believed was a stringent diet. The alter had had no interpersonal experiences since adolescence. A second woman, alluded to earlier, dissociated during the termination phase of therapy. Her alters had rarely emerged since she was removed from her abusive mother in mid-adolescence. Her discovery was prompted by weeping for which she was amnestic. This proved to be the weeping of a little girl alter who experienced termination as a repetition of her loss of her beloved father.

A 61-year-old man had spent over 30 years in unproductive therapy for depression and obsessive-compulsive neurosis. He had been tried on adequate doses of every available medication and had received trials of almost all major psychotherapies. After a year's treatment with no demonstrable results, he was screened for multiple personality disorder. All inquiries were negative. Inquiries repeated under hypnosis revealed multiple personality disorder. This individual was rigid and suffered mild cardiac and cerebral ischemic episodes on the basis of arteriosclerotic cardiovascular disease and a hypercoagulable state. His classic obsessive symptoms proved to reflect alters in conflict. For example, his undoing consisted of one alter's acting and another negating the action of the first. Obsessive thoughts were alters' harassing one another, and compulsions were made actions. Treatment was successful, and eliminated the "obsessional" phenomena. It was of note that over the years the alters' manifest differences had become quite attenuated. Their attitudes and memories remained very distinct, however.

A 72-year-old woman totally denied all dissociative symptomatology, but her multiple personality disorder daughter offered convincing documentation of the woman's condition. She sought help for an involutional depression. I noted a history of heart attacks and stroke. I also diagnosed and arranged for treatment of her diabetes mellitus. She was assessed for multiple personality disorder. An alter was found that admitted abusing the daughter, and spoke of its individuality diminishing over the last decade. The alter also had signs of depression. Tricyclics alleviated the affective component. Persistent mild signs of organicity were noted. At this point, the patient "confessed" her awareness of the multiple personality disorder, but declined active treatment. In subsequent reevaluations, it was clear that the alters were working toward communicating, and social improvements were notable. Unfortunately, organic impairment gradually increased. As her ego functions have been compromised, the alters have been unable to retain the segregation of their memories. At last assessment, the patient had separate entities, but their mental contents had few distinctions.

The last patient in this series was a woman who presented in an emergency ward a month before her 70th birthday, complaining she was possessed by a devil. Assessment disclosed mild organicity, a major depression, and signs suggestive of either an hallucinatory/delusional component or a possession-like form of multiple personality disorder. After tricyclics, it was clear the organicity was genuine rather than a depressive pseudodementia, and that the patient had multiple personality disorder. An alter, which also had mild organicity (but with a different voice and memory, purporting to be a demon), both imposed itself on the host via hallucinated threatening voices, and occasionally took over. I was told the patient had had psychotic depressions in which she berated herself for an affair her family was sure had not occurred. She was a pillar of the church. After inquiry, the following very incomplete account was reconstructed.

The patient had classic multiple personality disorder until her late 30s. In one alter, she had had an affair. This alter was largely suppressed. Over the next decade, the memory of the affair occasionally was recovered by the host, who felt very miserable and guilty. The demonic persecutor's criticism reached the host at those times. The resultant picture was of a psychotic depression. There were suicidal episodes and courses of electroconvulsive therapy (ECT). Over the passage of years, the alter that had the affair ceased to be separate. The patient now had one personality in chronic guilt over the affair, and the persecutor. She tried to confess her "sins," but was assured they were delusional. After tricyclics alleviated the depression's psychobiological components and the above history was elicited, psychotherapy was attempted. It was unsuccessful. Due to her organicity, the patient could neither comprehend nor maintain a therapeutic alliance. She got some relief from ventilating her guilt. After consultation with the family and clergy, an extrusive procedure described by Allison (36) was undertaken. It was successful. On six-year follow-up, the patient's organicity has progressed somewhat, and her depression begins to return if tricyclics are withdrawn for protracted periods. However, there has been no return of her multiple personality disorder. She has been happy and had peace of mind for the first time in nearly half a century.

These cases in older adults indicated that while some individuals' multiple personality disorder remains florid throughout their lives, in many there is a progressive diminution of the external manifestations, an atrophy of individual differences, and a spontaneous integration of some components during and after middle age.

These findings regarding initial presentations are supported by "second look" presentations; that is, patients whose multiple personality disorder was diagnosed, yet who declined treatment initially, and returned three to 10 years later. In brief, not a single patient in this group of 12 offered the same presentation that he or she had made before.

One patient seen on three occasions presented first as a neurotic depression, second as a paranoid schizophrenic, and finally as florid multiple personality disorder. In the first case, a neurasthenic depleted host was dominant for over a year. She was hospitalized when her depression worsened. When she returned, she heard voices arguing in her head and commenting critically on her actions, believed she was being followed, and appeared delusional. When she was seen again after a hospitalization for schizophrenia, she was seen as anxious, obsessional, and fearful of losing control. Her multiple personality disorder was discovered by her inclusion as a control case for a testing protocol.

A patient who presented with what appeared to be post-traumatic global amnesia after an accident was found to have multiple personality disorder during hypnotic exploration of her amnesia. After three years of displaying florid multiple personality disorder, she left treatment. On return, she presented in a depressed neurasthenic host amnestic for events between the accident and her regaining awareness. She complained of depression. She had shifted to a one alter dominant adaptation, but had several first-rank symptoms. She denied ever having had multiple personality disorder. The alter that sought help was previously unknown to me, as was I to her.

Two patients who dissociated rapidly and floridly in front of me as teenagers returned for treatment in their mid-20s. One had repressed all recollection of her multiple personality disorder, which now was restricted to alters covertly influencing the host. She denied all classic symptoms and amnesia, but was positive for several first rank passive influence symptoms. The second had evolved so that more and more alters passed as one. The only external difference maintained was that male alters wore slacks. A helper personality called for an appointment, explained how things had changed in the interim, and said all alters now agreed to be in treatment.

A woman with florid multiple personality disorder returned after eight years with some alters desperately trying to suppress the manifestations of alters. While before she was "textbook classic," she now presented a chronic picture of battles for dominance, with rare moments in which one alter predominated clearly. Another patient returned after seven years. In the interim, the insights gained in a single session held before her husband curtailed treatment had eroded the separateness of her only other personality. Most of its memories were recovered by the other through dreams and diary-writing. As this occurred, the alter became less distinct and ceased to emerge.

The case of "Cissy" is an instructive example. At age 16, she was seen for a single interview. She was an emancipated minor and single parent, already overwhelmed by life before she was gang-raped, and feared she would "freak out." As I took her history, I was impressed with her rapidly changing facies and voice, with her frequent requests that I repeat questions, and with her giving answers several minutes later to questions that she had not responded to originally. My initial impression was that the patient was on drugs, was psychotic, or both. As the interview progressed, I called attention to her evasion of all questions about her family. At this point, voice and facies switched, and the patient said, "Cissy don't know anything about that." I made no intrusive inquiry, but began to consider multiple personality disorder. A few minutes later, as I asked about the rape, another abrupt change occurred. "That will never happen to her again. You keep your hands to yourself or I'll cut you bad." The entity that spoke moved to a far corner of the office and pulled out but did not open a large knife. In the ensuing dialogue, this entity identified itself as "Maria." In a few minutes, "Cissy" reemerged, dazed and stunned, to find the knife in her hands. "Cissy" made another appointment, but did not appear. When I called by phone, the "Maria" voice said she would not return.

In the intervening seven years, I received several requests for information on the patient from physicians and agencies. All were politely skeptical of my report. At first, these professionals saw the patient as suffering schizophrenia, a borderline state, or hysteria. Then the requests came from general physicians, who were seeing the patient for somatic distresses, including migraine and irritable bowel syndrome.

In time, "Cissy" became stable. She worked and got married. She sought help from a rape victims' group. As treatment began, she began to have dreams and then recollections of incest experiences, which she tried to suppress. She entered an incest survivors' group in an alter, "Alice," who passed for "Cissy" but had recollections of the incest. Several alters, co-conscious and troubled by the incest, attended the group, which included multiple personality disorder patients. No one suspected her of multiple personality disorder. Finally, the co-conscious alters decided to call me. They had decided to work to integrate. They confided in the group's leader, and then the group, and received warm support for their plans.

The patient who presented for treatment was calm, poised, and collected. She said she was "Alice," but that she and the others passed for "Cissy" and found that most convenient. After three or four years of florid dissociation and fugues, during which they wandered about dazed and were subject to further assaults, a group of alters had gradually won over the others to pass as one and remain co-conscious, except when alone. That process had not been smooth. For some years, this had been a struggle, resulting in numerous somatic manifestations of conflict and transient "psychotic" episodes. In the last year, however, all had agreed to work to be well and to integrate, although they could not imagine such a process. Their own efforts to join had proven inadequate. "Alice" said their marriage, new children, and their sense from the groups "that therapy could work" made them motivated for help. This has proven to be the case.

In summary, the natural history of multiple personality disorder involves most individuals' making very different presentations over the course of their patient careers. It is uncommon for a patient to remain in a florid publicly observable dissociated condition on an ongoing basis.

THOUGHTS ON THE MANIFEST APPEARANCE OF MULTIPLE PERSONALITY DISORDER

A review of the observations and data presented above leads me to conclude that what is essential to multiple personality disorder across its many presentations is no more than the presence, within an individual, of more than one structured entity with a sense of its own existence. Such entities are, by tradition, called personalities. However, the term "personality" may imply a higher degree of elaborateness than is consistent with clinical reality in certain cases, and imply as well that such complexity is essential to the condition. Braun has developed a list of terms to describe different degrees of complexity in such entities (3, 28). Observational data of such patients and the explorations undertaken in their therapies indicate that definitions and criteria based on behavioral evidence may misrepresent multiple personality disorder as it actually occurs. While the details of any definition or diagnostic criteria are a matter for professional consensus, it is clear that most patients who satisfy DSM-III criteria for multiple personality disorder at some points in time do not satisfy such criteria at others.

Multiple personality disorder appears to develop as a dissociative defense in the face of overwhelming childhood events. The raison d'etre of multiple personality disorder is to provide a structured dissociative defense against overwhelming traumata and the possible repetition of the same or analogous traumata. The emitted observable manifestations of multiple personality disorder are epiphenomena and tools of the defensive purpose. In terms of the patient's needs, the personalities need only be as distinct, public, and elaborate as becomes necessary in the handling of stressful situations. In childhood cases, investment in separateness and distinctness is usually minimal. Anything further results from hypertrophy or secondary autonomy of these processes, and from whatever narcissistic investments and secondary gains become associated with them. While adult cases' personalities usually have considerable autonomy and investment in separateness, they may or may not, in the course of performing their functions and achieving their missions, appear to need to develop or show their differences. In short, what is essential to multiple personality disorder is what is already found in childhood cases.

For research purposes, then, it is useful to rely on DSM-III diagnostic criteria to assure that the patients being studied clearly demonstrate the classic phenomena of multiple personality disorder at the time at which the research endeavors are undertaken. For clinical purposes, however, a strict reliance on DSM-III criteria will probably perpetuate the delayed diagnosis and misdiagnosis of patients with multiple personality disorder.

It may be useful to review patients' statements relevant to the manifestness of their multiple personality disorder, along with insights gained in the course of treatment. Patient and therapist observations concur that the resiliency of the host personality, that personality in ostensible control of the body most of the time over a period of time (3), is a major determinant. If the host is fairly robust, relatively few external stimuli will overwhelm it and prompt the emergence of specialized alters. Furthermore, a powerful host, resilient in the face of stressors, may be able to suppress others for long periods. If such an arrangement is fairly stable, there may be no overt evidence of multiple personality disorder for many years on end. It stands to reason that in many patients, the openness of their multiple personality disorder may fluctuate with the degree of stress in their lives.

Another dimension relates to the personalities' degree of cooperation. If it is high, they may share contemporary memory, pass for one another, and come out smoothly in tandem to help with problem areas. Such cases show neither amnesia nor manifest differences. If cooperation is high, but clandestine and unknown to the host, the most one will find is subtle evidence of one alter's influencing another; that is, some of the passive influence first-rank symptoms. If the alters are in conflict and contention, but their battles lead to no clear-cut victories, the patient, his clinical picture dominated by signs of such battles, may appear borderline or psychotic. If alters in conflict succeed in replacing one another in control, one sees overt multiple personality disorder. Hence, issues of power and relative strength among alters influence the clinical presentation.

A related dimension is the way the personalities learn to influence one another. If they do so by inner dialogue, a cooperative common front may be seen. If they do so covertly, or manipulatively, passive influence phenomena are seen in an apparently unified individual. If they do so by inner verbalized threats, a hallucinated quasi-psychotic picture may be found. If they do so by assuming complete executive control, full multiple personality disorder will be seen.

Another dimension is secrecy. Sometimes personalities choose to keep their existence hidden; sometimes powerful alters suppress others. Under such circumstances, patients usually know of, but disavow, their multiple personality disorder, and do not answer diagnostic questions with candor.

Commonality of motivation may unify otherwise diverse alters for a long period of time, causing them to collaborate. A common reason for this is child-rearing. When the motivation ceases to be shared, overt difference may emerge. The author has seen many patients whose florid multiple personality disorder subsided with childbirth, and became open again when the children went to school or reached adolescence.

Alters' investment in separateness is a self-evident dimension with regard to the degree to which the multiple personality disorder will be manifest. It is my experience that for about 90 percent of multiple personality disorder patients, this investment is in the personal sense of separateness rather than in achieving its recognition by others. Hospitalized multiple personality disorder patients whose diagnoses are challenged are prone to make a show of separateness to try to convince others of their diagnosis (a move that usually backfires); but this is an iatrogenic phenomenon. Patients should never be forced to "prove" that their distress is legitimate.

Patients who come to see their condition as an asset, who have

circumstances favoring strong secondary gain, who bring a creative flair to everything in their lives, or who have found that the
creation of further alters serves as an outlet for unacceptable affects
(or as an ad hoc solution to intrapsychic conflict) are likely to be
quite overt. In contrast, patients who hate or are ashamed of their
disorder, who feel it encumbers their lives, who are not inclined to
invest special creativity in each endeavor, or who experience the
creation of alters as traumatic, are likely to be quite subdued.

It is commonplace for multiple personality disorder to become
more overt and clearly expressed as patients are diagnosed and
enter therapy. Often, the patient, the doctor, and concerned others
concur that circumstances appear to deteriorate as treatment gets
under way. This leads to concerns about the creation or reinforcement of pathology. In actuality, beginning treatment initiates a
major disequilibrium in most multiple personality disorder patients (32). Previous homeostatic devices are disturbed, the mechanism of dissociation (a powerful defense) is brought under scru-
tiny, traumatic material is uncovered, and negative therapeutic
reactions are common. It is difficult to conceive of a more
uncomfortable and demanding therapy.

In connection with these discomforts, the alters often are
remobilized to once again defend against the pain of the past, and
prevent its being reexperienced in the therapy. As the host's
function is compromised by the eroding of amnestic barriers, its
resilience and functional abilities may diminish, encouraging
both the reemergence of alters who attend to specialized functions,
and the intercession of helper personalities. Punitive alters who
forbid anger against abusers or the sharing of information on abuse
escalate their punitive behaviors. For these, and many other
reasons as well, such apparent "flowering" of overt multiple
personality disorder is a natural consequence of its treatment, and
can be anticipated, much as moments of regression and acting out
may be encountered in any intense change-oriented psychotherapy. The excellent outcomes of multiple personality disorder
treatments in which these phenomena are noted further suggests
that these events are often concomitants of the therapeutic process
(7, 26, 32).

CONCLUSION

The classic manifestations of multiple personality disorder are best understood as one of several phases in the natural history of multiple personality disorder. In most patients, this particular phase is not invariably predominant over the longitudinal time course of their lives. Instead, it is seen intermittently. An appreciation of the many other forms in which multiple personality disorder may manifest itself is essential to an understanding of the problems surrounding its underdiagnosis and misdiagnosis, and may, in time, contribute to resolving some of the controversies that surround this clinical condition.

References

1. Kluft RP: Casefinding for multiple personality. The diagnosis and treatment of multiple personality in a community mental health center. Paper presented at the Annual Meeting of the American Psychiatric Association, Atlanta, May, 1978

2. Kluft RP: Epidemiology of multiple personality. Paper presented at the Annual Meeting of the American Psychiatric Association, Chicago, May, 1979

3. Kluft RP: An introduction to multiple personality disorder. Psychiatric Annals 14:19-24, 1984

4. American Psychiatric Association: Diagnostic and Statistical Manual of Mental Disorders (Third Edition). Washington, DC, American Psychiatric Association, 1980

5. Putnam FW, Post RM, Guroff JJ, et al: 100 cases of multiple personality disorder. Presented at the Annual Meeting of the American Psychiatric Association, as New Research Abstract #77, New York, 1983

6. Kluft RP: Multiple personality in childhood. Psychiatr Clin North Am 7:121-134, 1984

7. Kluft RP: Treatment of multiple personality disorder: a study of 33 cases. Psychiatr Clin North Am 7:9-29, 1984

8. Kluft RP: Hypnotherapy of childhood multiple personality disorder. Am J Clin Hypn (in press)

9. Kluft RP, Braun BG, Sachs RG: Multiple personality, intrafamilial abuse, and family psychiatry. International Journal of Family Psychiatry (in press)

10. Fagan J, McMahon P: Incipient multiple personality in children: four cases. J Nerv Ment Dis 172:26-36, 1984

11. Kluft RP: Varieties of hypnotic interventions in the treatment of multiple personality. Am J Clin Hypn 24:230-240, 1982

12. Coons PM: The differential diagnosis of multiple personality: a comprehensive review. Psychiatr Clin North Am 7:51-67, 1984

13. Bliss EL: Multiple personalities: a report of 14 cases with implications for schizophrenia and hysteria. Arch Gen Psychiatry 37:1388-1397, 1980

14. Ellenberger HF: The Discovery of the Unconscious. New York, Basic Books, 1970

15. Ward W, Farrelli L: The Healing of Lia. New York, Macmillan Publishing Co., 1982

16. Braun BG: Hypnosis creates multiple personality: myth or reality? International Journal of Clinical and Experimental Hypnosis 32:191-197, 1984

17. Kluft RP: The presentation of multiple personality disorder, in Multiple Personality and Dissociation. Edited by Braun BG, Kluft RP. New York, Guilford Press (in press)

18. Kluft RP: The psychophysiology of multiple personality disorder: analytic perspectives. Paper presented at the Annual Meeting of the American Psychiatric Association, Los Angeles, May, 1984

19. Horevitz RP, Braun BG: Are multiple personalities borderline? An analysis of 33 cases. Psychiatr Clin North Am 7:69-87, 1984

20. Clary WF, Burstin KJ, Carpenter JS: Multiple personality and borderline personality disorder. Psychiatr Clin North Am 7:89-99, 1984

21. Gruenewald D: Multiple personality and splitting phenomena: a reconceptualization. J Nerv Ment Dis 164:385-393, 1977

22. Spiegel D: Multiple personality as a post-traumatic stress disorder. Psychiatr Clin North Am 7:101-110, 1984

23. Erickson MH, Kubie L: The permanent relief of an obsessional phobia: by means of communication with an unsuspected dual personality. Psychoanal Q 8:38-51, 1939

24. Kluft RP: Diagnosing multiple personality disorder. Pennsylvania Medicine 87:44-46, 1984

25. Mellor CS: First rank symptoms in schizophrenia. Br J Psychiatry 117:15-23, 1970

26. Kluft RP: Hypnotherapeutic crisis intervention in multiple personality. Am J Clin Hypn 26:73-83, 1983

27. Bliss EL: Multiple personalities, related disorders, and hypnosis. Am J Clin Hypn 26:114-123, 1983

28. Braun BG: Neurophysiologic changes in multiple personality due to integration: a preliminary report. Am J Clin Hypn 26:84-92, 1983

29. Putnam FW, Loewenstein RJ, Silberman EK, et al: Multiple personality disorder in a hospital setting. J Clin Psychiatry 45:172-175, 1984

30. Coons PM: Multiple personality: diagnostic considerations. J Clin Psychiatry 41:330-336, 1980

31. Greaves GB: Multiple personality: 165 years after Mary Reynolds. J Nerv Ment Dis 168:577-596, 1980

32. Kluft RP: Aspects of the treatment of multiple personality disorder. Psychiatric Annals 14:51-55, 1984

33. Braun BG: Psychophysiologic phenomena in multiple personality and hypnosis. Am J Clin Hypn 26:124-137, 1983

34. Spiegel H, Spiegel D: Trance and Treatment: Clinical Uses of Hypnosis. New York, Basic Books, 1978

35. Bliss EL, Larson EM, Nakashima SR: Auditory hallucinations and schizophrenia. J Nerv Ment Dis 171:30-33, 1983

36. Allison RB: A new treatment approach for multiple personalities. Am J Clin Hypn 17:15-32, 1974

10

Discussion: A Clinician's Perspective

Richard E. Hicks, M.D.

10

Discussion: A Clinician's Perspective

The need to escape from pain in its myriad physical and emotional forms is one of the basic biologically rooted characteristics of the human organism. Sandler and Joffe, in their thoughtful 1969 discussion of intrapsychic adaptation, propose that the need for a basic feeling of safety, encompassing a sense of both physical and psychological integrity, is the prime motivating force in human behavior (1). They propose further that if the basic feeling of safety cannot be maintained within tolerable limits by means that serve the purpose of adaptation within the realms of both external (extrapsychic) and internal (intrapsychic) reality, adaptation in the former will be sacrificed in the interest of preserving adaptation in the latter. In other words, if we are unable to create a real situation that we can tolerate, we will, within the limits of our individual capacities, create, intrapsychically, the illusion of a more tolerable reality.

It is our current level of understanding that those persons who, in adulthood, function as multiple personalities, have, earlier in life, found themselves helpless to change an emotionally intolerable reality. Depending upon the age of the child at the time of the overwhelming traumatization, and upon the frequency and duration of the traumatic experiences, there is probably either a failure to establish a unified personal identity (with the continuation of multiple self-representations, some of which achieve sufficient organization to be thought of as personalities) or the later dissociation of complexes of components of the existing psychic structure, so that a previously unified personal identity is sacrificed in the interest of intrapsychic adaptation (that is, trying to feel as safe as possible under the circumstances).

The above, although compatible with numerous clinical observations, remains highly speculative. We do not really know at what age an adult with multiple personality disorder may have become diagnosable, nor exactly how the disorder develops intrapsychically. Kluft and others contributing to this monograph have cautioned that the patient's retrospective reports do not constitute definitive scientific evidence for the age at which their dissociative condition developed. Most patients' accounts are plausible in the main. At times, confirmation of allegations is possible. But their overall credibility may be unfairly compromised by the presence of unlikely minor components, a form of elaboration encountered in many cases.

It does seem reasonable to assume some degree of historical inaccuracy when, for instance, a 40-year-old patient reports the presence of a prenatal personality that she believes to have become separate before birth. I have heard such reports from two adult patients. Still, based on the accumulated experience of an increasing number of clinicians and researchers, we are probably correct in believing that there are both internal and external determinants for most manifestations of multiple personality disorder, and that most patients with multiple personality disorder experienced the initial external determinants of their disorders quite early in life. We also are probably correct in assuming that most multiple personality disorder patients experienced the onset of their illness in either prelatency or latency. Just how early or how late in life multiple personality disorder can develop is not known. The diagnosis has been made in patients ranging from three years of age to just under 70.

Similarly, we do not know the incidence of multiple personality disorder in the general population. At present, those patients found to suffer multiple personality disorder often have been misdiagnosed for many years (see Chapters 4, 8, and 9 of this monograph). We have no way to estimate how many patients with multiple personality disorder never receive correct diagnosis and treatment. Putnam states that 1,000 current multiple personality disorder patients have been identified in North America. Frischholz reports that the 92 scientific contributors to the First International Conference on Multiple Personality and Dissociative States, held in 1984, collectively accounted for over 400 documented cases of multiple personality disorder seen in the last decade. This is an impressive figure, especially in view of the fact that many of the 360 who attended the conference but did not present papers had also seen one or more multiple personality disorder patients over the same period. Some of us, who were in practice many years before we began to recognize the existence of multiple personality disorder, have come to perceive that our long-standing prior failure to recognize multiple personality disorder, even when face to face with it in the therapeutic situation, has been a significant research-worthy clinical and public health phenomenon in itself, with manifold external and internal determinants (see Chapters 1, 8, and 9 of this monograph).

Multiple personality disorder is the current great imitator of other psychiatric, physical, and neurological disorders. The patient may present as depressed or bizarre, psychotic, catatonic (with or without waxy flexibility); or in status epilepticus, as severely compulsive or sociopathic; as mentally retarded, or with a somatic memory in the form of psychogenic pain, with some amenorrhea or dysmenorrhea; with chaotic relationships, or panic attacks; with headaches, paranoid delusions, psychosexual disorders, blackouts, substance abuse, self-mutilation, hypomania, explosive outbursts, conversion symptoms, phobic reactions, kleptomania, hallucinations, manipulative suicide attempts, and genuine suicide attempts. This list is representative, and not intended to be exhaustive by any means. Any one multiple personality disorder patient may present with any or all of the above clinical signs and symptoms among his or her system of different personalities. In fact, each of the above represents the manifest symptomatology of one or more of my first diagnosed multiple personality disorder patient's several personalities.

PERSONAL EXPERIENCE

When this particular patient initially came to see me, she was a competent-appearing young woman who was working fairly successfully as a psychiatric nurse. The presenting personality did not reveal to me, nor did she even know, that in her off-duty hours another personality was working as a prostitute and using fair amounts of "speed" and other illicit drugs. Nor did she reveal that in the 10 preceding years she had been hospitalized 20 times under 12 different psychiatric diagnoses and had been treated with eight antipsychotics, three tricyclic antidepressants, electroconvulsive therapy (ECT), lithium carbonate, three antianxiety drugs, four anticonvulsant drugs, and prolonged individual and group psychotherapy with five different therapists (four psychiatrists and one nurse practitioner). Five months later she was hospitalized and had an extensive evaluation for status epilepticus with atypical grand mal seizures (discovered one year later to be a manifestation of rage by one of her sixty-six alternate personalities).

Following neurologic, metabolic, and endocrinologic evaluations in a general hospital, she was transferred to my service in a psychiatric hospital. Her behavior had become alternately: hostile and demanding; fearful, tearful, and shaking; or depressed and suicidal. Two months later she led us to suspect her correct diagnosis when she told a nurse she was really someone with a name different from the one we knew her by, and that there were five others with her as well. There is no telling how much longer she would have remained misdiagnosed if she had not revealed herself. If I had known then what I know now about multiple personality disorder, I believe that the signs she showed early in treatment probably would have alerted me to consider this diagnosis as a serious possibility three to four months earlier, and to have made the diagnosis with certainty within her first month of hospitalization.

Since that time, 7½ years ago, I have worked intensively with six more multiple personality disorder patients and participated in making the diagnosis in 15 others, including a 10-year-old fire-setter. I have also seen four patients in whom I suspected the diagnosis, but was unable, for various reasons, to determine with certainty whether multiple personality disorder was present. I assessed three other patients whom others thought might have multiple personality disorder. In these instances, I did not find evidence to demonstrate that the condition was present.

To the best of my and my colleagues' recollections, during a period of over 20 years prior to 1977, only three staff psychiatrists at the hospital in which I practice had even seen a patient with multiple personality disorder. As of this writing, five of the 20 hospital-based attending psychiatrists are actively treating seven multiple personality disorder patients, five of whom are inpatients; and two of 10 psychiatry residents are each treating one outpatient with multiple personality disorder.

Most of the psychiatrists and other mental health professionals I have met who have diagnosed and treated patients with multiple personality disorder have found little initial support from their colleagues. Some have found the going very difficult. Many have been told, in various ways, by their colleagues, their supervisors, and others, that they were simply wrong, that there was no such thing as multiple personality disorder; or, if the diagnosis was considered accurate, that it was probably basically a seizure disorder or an affective disorder and should be treated primarily with medication. Worse, many have experienced quite derisive criticism or ridicule, either directly or indirectly. In one instance a member of a nursing staff told a multiple personality disorder patient that the patient's doctor was crazy and diagnosed everyone as having multiple personality disorder.

Certainly, multiple personality disorder evokes some very strong emotions. I know of no other illness that stimulates such strong denials of the possibility of its existence, and an absence of interest in many very capable clinicians who have very intense spontaneous curiosity about other clinical phenomena.

DISCUSSION OF CHAPTERS

Why should this be so? In Chapter 1 of this monograph, Dr. Goodwin speaks eloquently to this question. It is indeed difficult for us to believe our patients when they report such things as sadistic, ritualistic torture at meetings of various cults, or their sale by their upper-middle class parents to groups of upper-middle class men for sexual orgies, or their use for the production of babies for sale on the illegal market. We are, as Dr. Goodwin says, "incredulous" when we hear and see a patient reliving, while dissociated into a child personality, her preparation with a dildo at age two for intercourse with a parent and others at age three. Unfortunately, we have tended to be incredulous upon hearing of much less extensive abuse and exploitation. A current news item indicates that 200,000 instances of child abuse were reported nationally last year.

Dr. Goodwin's extremely well informed explanations of incredulity on the part of mental health professionals (applicable as well to the general population) are quite within the realm of good clinical interpretation based on the evidence at hand. I would like to emphasize some points and offer a few additional thoughts.

Dr. Goodwin makes reference to a relatively frequent phenomenon: the false retraction of accusations previously made by victims of abuse. This has its counterpart in the course of the treatment of many multiple personality disorder patients. Just when some of the family's secrets of abuses are about to surface or have been revealed but have not yet been worked through, many patients attempt to deny the presence of multiple personality disorder and retract the newly revealed secrets. They often go on to say they have "made it all up" for the purposes of "gaining attention."

With regard to the relationship between familial and professional denial or disbelief and the development of dissociative mechanisms, these, at the very least, reinforce and encourage dissociation and repression. In the treatment of adult patients with various forms of dissociative and conversion symptomatology, and in work with borderline conditions as well, I have found that some individuals who were abused as children were repeatedly admonished that they were lying, or were told they had imagined or dreamed the abuse experiences. In other instances, the abuses were acknowledged (at least to some extent) but were treated as insignificant or were blamed on the victim. These child victims were then obliged, both because of these external pressures and forces within themselves, to disbelieve their own vivid perceptions.

Dr. Goodwin has noted the extreme infrequency of false accusations of abuse made by children against adults. There is an increasing number of confirmations from sources other than multiple personality disorder patients themselves of the abuses they have experienced. The problem is that these are scattered among a fairly large number of therapists, and the data have not yet been formally collected and analyzed. In any one person's practice such confirmations are not frequent, although there are frequently strongly suggestive kinds of evidence, such as parents who deny everything and avoid any contact with their grown child's therapist during years of treatment, or parents who deny nothing while also confirming nothing, as if standing on their "fifth amendment" rights against self-incrimination.

On more than one occasion, I have had the opportunity to have a patient's previously repressed or dissociated memories of severe abuses confirmed by independent sources. Based on this experience, I cannot overemphasize the importance for health professionals to believe patients who report past abuses or recover memories of them; and the importance for mental health professionals to lead the way toward helping them, when the evidence points in that direction, to recognize the deceptions and injustices to which they have been subjected, despite their sometimes prolonged disbelief. It is necessary to be especially alert when the patient's perceptions of the parents are "too good to be true," given the clinical picture. For example, if a patient either has multiple personality disorder or, in the absence of that diagnosis, has amnesia for large segments of life between ages five or six and the late teens or early 20s with no other available explanation, it is plausible to consider the probability that the patient has been traumatized. If the patient's family is then described in very positive terms, and the family denies knowledge of any significant traumata to the patient, it is reasonable to assume a high probability that either they did not know (raising the question of why they would not) or, more likely, that they know and are hiding the truth.

There are several possibilities I would like to add to Dr. Goodwin's discussion of the incredulity of professionals about the existence of multiple personality disorder, which, as noted previously, sometimes is accompanied by very strong negative feelings. First, the existence of multiple personality disorder may be perceived as an assault on the concept "person," which is a concept that is deeply ingrained and cherished by all of us. Although we may recognize "personhood" to be extremely complex and highly variable, there is one thing about which most of us became certain early in our lives: that a "person" is a singular individual being with a singular individual identity. Even the individual personalities of the multiple personality disorder patient believe in their wholeness and separateness, physically and psychologically. Identity as a separate whole person is a highly prized possession.

When we work with patients with multiple personality disorder, our sense of reality is challenged. At the level of our sensory perceptions, the patient has a single human body; but it appears to be the vehicle for the behavior (or "lives") of extremely different persons, many of whom may not even know each other. We have stepped "behind the looking glass" into a world in which major aspects of reality are governed by primary process. We find it necessary to form separate relationships with separate personalities, as if they were truly separate people. We cannot even identify one personality as the person who is the patient. Especially if there are many personalities, intense affects, and frequent switches, it can be very disconcerting. It is strange, uncanny, and all too "unbelievable."

In addition, the plight of the multiple personality disorder patient may serve as a reminder of the fragility of our own state of being, not only as individuals with singular identities, but also as persons with continuous lives. Perhaps empathy with their lack of singular identity and the apparent discontinuity of their lives may be perceived unconsciously as a personal threat to the interviewer's sense of his or her own self and existence, similar to the fear of death. We are familiar with the common tendency to avoid the terminally ill. A colleague once admonished me that in suggesting the possibility of multiple personality disorder in a patient, I was raising the possibility of diagnosing "a malignancy." This poignant choice of expression reflects the depths of aversion some feel toward this diagnosis.

Finally, accounts of multiple personality disorder, from early on, have depicted the switching of personalities as a means by which to give free reign to the most forbidden impulses. The Jekyll-Hyde dichotomy is a paradigm for a general impression of what multiple personality disorder is about: a person who is an otherwise upright citizen, much as ourselves, yet has no control over his or her becoming a sadistic monster. Aspects of ourselves that we are protected from by our own highly invested defensive systems are, in the Jekyll-Hyde paradigm, capable of overcoming the conscious "good self" and gaining unbridled access to consciousness and action. That is all well and good in fiction, but it may be perceived as a great threat, especially at an unconscious level, if we recognize this literary stereotype as a real possibility for enactment by the multiple personality disorder patient before us.

Repressed conflictual aggression and sadism are universal, even in people who are healthy enough to be able to repress or sublimate these impulses. Child abuse and multiple personality disorder may reflect, too vividly for some, their own personal experiences or unconscious impulses, and fears about them, requiring rejection without due consideration.

In Chapter 2 of this monograph, Dr. Wilbur cites the general categories of child abuse experiences: nonnurturing, sexual abuse, physiological abuse, psychological abuse, and physical abuse. She indicated that experiences within these categories, or combinations of them, can be etiologically significant in the formation of all forms of psychogenic illness. It has been my impression, (perhaps skewed by a predominance of such patients in my practice for many years) that child abuse, in any and all of these forms, is an especially common etiological factor in most severe forms of character pathology, such as various forms of borderline and narcissistic disorders, as well as multiple personality disorder.

Dr. Wilbur indicates that the nature of specific alternate personalities is shaped by the nature of the traumatic situations to which the child has been subjected, including the specific forms of abuse, overwhelming affects that resulted, and the character of the abuser (as in the example of the stepfather who could be intimidated by the child's brandishing a knife). Dr. Wilbur describes alternates whose characters and functions serve to preserve and express drives or sublimatory activities, and still others whose characters and functions are based on identification with the aggressor. Implicit in these descriptions are additional functions of alternate personalities: partial repetitions of the earlier traumas, reenactments, revenge, pathological gratifications of masochistic and narcissistic needs resulting from developmental arrests or fixations, and the obtaining of secondary gains. All of these, as Dr. Wilbur has indicated, basically occur in the interest of survival. Dr. Wilbur offers a very concise model for the formation of multiple personality disorder, emphasizing the central role of the patient's intense aggression, which in the adult patients I have seen has regularly been of murderous proportions.

The formation of alternates, at one level, is an escape from unbearable pain and anxiety. But alternates also serve the need to escape from the patient's own unacceptable impulses, such as the rage that might otherwise erupt and result in violent, aggressive acts. Occasionally an alter embodying such feelings escapes control and acts upon them, through assault, rape, murder, or suicide. Dr. Wilbur discusses the origin of hysterical and psychosomatic symptoms in specific intrapsychic conflicts that have been localized in individual alternates. She then goes on to discuss the tragic consequences of child abuse that are inherent in the lives of most multiple personality disorder patients, resulting in part from the blindness of society to the abuses. We are only beginning to recognize the extent to which, as a society, we have failed to acknowledge the extent of this problem. Finally, Dr. Wilbur recommends the importance of a readiness "to appreciate, understand, and listen to the communications of infants, children, and adolescents," which includes careful observation and interpretation of both the nonverbal and verbal aspects of their communications, as a step in the direction of prevention.

In the course of their contributions, Drs. Braun and Sachs in Chapter 3, Mr. Frischholz in Chapter 5, and Dr. Braun in Chapter 6, present accounts of the history and current conceptualizations of dissociation and hypnosis, and their relationship to multiple personality disorder. Current conceptualizations, based largely on studies of hypnosis, strongly suggest that both hypnosis and multiple personality disorder are dependent upon the capacity of the subject to dissociate. It is postulated that persons who use dissociation as the "defense mechanism of choice" for defense against the overwhelming affects associated with psychic trauma have a higher genetically determined capacity for dissociation than persons who respond to such traumata with nondissociative defenses.

An alternative explanation, however, requires consideration. It is possible that dependence on the dissociative defense might be determined less by a genetically heightened capacity for dissociation than by the unavailability of sufficiently developed other defense mechanisms. We do not really know whether differences in the capacity to dissociate may be present to approximately the same degree in most or all infants; but we do know that it is capable of being more or less inhibited by early developmental factors that usually lead to the substitution of other defenses in response to traumatic experiences. Such a plausible formulation can be elaborated from current object relations theory. Fortunately, this is a highly theoretical question and is not crucial to the most pressing of current problems in relation to multiple personality disorder, namely, learning to recognize and treat it.

The remainder of Chapter 3 offers an excellent discussion of the process of the development of multiple personality disorder within the framework of "predisposing, precipitating, and perpetuating factors." It is completely compatible with Kluft's four factor theory (2). I would offer qualifications about only three statements: 1) that, "In order to promote the development of multiple personality disorder, the abuse must be frequent, unpredictable, and inconsistent"; 2) that, "Infrequent maltreatment will lead to sporadic dissociative episodes that do not take on a life history of their own"; and 3) that, "The child is also exposed to some form of love." These are statements that I believe are usually applicable to the development of multiple personality disorder, but not invariably so. Some room should be left open for exceptions. Drs. Braun and Sachs' discussion of the transition of the dissociative defense in multiple personality disorder from an adaptive one in childhood to a maladaptive one when carried into adulthood, is an excellent example of the Sandler and Joffe (1) hypothesis regarding the sacrifice of adaptation in the external world in the interest of an intrapsychic adaptation. It is characteristic for some of a multiple personality disorder patient's alternates to be hyperalert and overreactive to any cue that might be the least bit suggestive of a recurrence of earlier traumatic experiences, either in fact or through vivid, painful memories. For such alternates there is little or no discrimination between past and present, and similarities are perceived not as being similar but as being identical, due to the predominance of primary process thinking in such alternates.

The example of the shift of the multiple personality disorder defense from adaptive in childhood to maladaptive in adulthood stimulates some thoughts about a possible relationship to the characteristic delay that we believe exists between the childhood onset and the adult diagnosis of multiple personality disorder. One possibility this suggests is that while the multiple personality disorder defense is serving a truly adaptive function vis-a-vis actual ongoing traumatic experiences, usually intrafamilial abuse, the internalized representations of the traumatizers are not as likely to be indiscriminately projected onto other relationships. Rather, this is more likely to occur after the multiple personality disorder patient has left the abusive family, and it results in a manifestly less adaptive individual. This explanation, if correct, would be only one of many for the hiatus between onset and diagnosis (see Chapters 8 and 9 of this monograph).

We are in debt to Dr. Putnam for his extensive literature review of the dissociative disorders in Chapter 4 of this monograph, which demonstrates a clear consensus, derived from many studies in varied contexts, that, " . . . in most patients the precipitation of a dissociative reaction is associated with substantial psychological stress or traumatic experiences." It is also of interest that for the three most severe forms of dissociative disorders—psychogenic amnesia, psychogenic fugue, and multiple personality disorder—a childhood history of a disturbed home situation or child-parent relationship has been cited as a "significant" predisposing factor.

Mr. Frischholz, in a carefully written chapter, traces the development of the concept of dissociation from its initial psychological application to multiple personality disorder, nearly a century ago; and he leads us through the implications of certain difficulties in its definition and acceptance as a psychological mechanism, along with the similar difficulties undergone by the concept of multiple personality disorder. He outlines the confusion created by classic dissociation theory's "criterion of noninterference" and explains its inappropriateness as a test for the presence of dissociation, as, for instance, with regard to the question of whether hypnosis is a form of dissociation.

Mr. Frischholz adheres at present to a generic definition of dissociation; that is, "to dissociate means to sever the association of one thing from another," and indicates, in effect, that there is no generally accepted metapsychological definition of dissociation, nor of its relationship to other defense mechanisms, especially repression. I can only agree with what I perceive to be Frischholz's wish that we might all agree to return to efforts to learn what dissociation is, phenomenologically, metapsychologically and, perhaps one day, neurophysiologically, through the study of its major clinical manifestation, multiple personality disorder.

Noting that " . . . there is (also) no universally agreed upon definition of (hypnosis)," he goes on to review questions concerning hypnosis and multiple personality disorder that have been researched experimentally and in controlled studies. These indicate the following, as I interpret the material presented: that not everyone is hypnotizable and that there are differences in hypnotizability that tend to be fairly consistent across various tests; that people who have been abused as children produce significantly higher mean hypnotizability scores than people who were not abused, as do patients with multiple personality disorder when compared to nonmultiple personality disorder patients and normals; that highly hypnotizable subjects, including untreated multiple personality disorder patients, experience the "hidden observer" phenomenon at the rate of approximately 50 percent of subjects, but that more research is needed to fully understand the implications of the phenomenon for hypnosis and dissociation; that a genetic factor for hypnotizability has been hypothesized, but that there is to date only one twin study, and in that study, " . . . the higher correlations between the hypnotizability scores of monozygotic twins than among dizygotic twins or other family members," were not high enough (or low enough) to be conclusive; that the capacity for imaginative involvement, while correlating with hypnotizability, may prove to be determined by either environmental or genetic factors; and, that certain observations of behavioral response currently used in hypnotizability scales have been challenged, and may prove inadequate to test for changes in volitional control during hypnosis.

In Chapter 6, Dr. Braun presents a study testing the null hypothesis of the transgenerational occurrence of multiple personality disorder (the null hypothesis stating that there is no transgenerational occurrence). He demonstrates clearly that there is an occurrence of multiple personality disorder across generations, even if we were to accept only those cross-generational cases of multiple personality disorder satisfying the stringent diagnostic criteria of Braun's category 4 (that is, confirmed). Braun notes the methodological limitations of his study, which prevent further conclusions. Additional studies will be necessary to determine the statistical significance of this occurrence and especially to determine the factors responsible for it. Nevertheless, along with the fact that five (27.7 percent) of the 18 multiple personality disorder patients' mothers or stepmothers had a certainty rating of 4 for multiple personality disorder (that is, confirmed), it is impressive to see that of the three instances in which one of the index cases' children received a multiple personality disorder rating of 4, in two instances the child's other parent was also confirmed to have multiple personality disorder; and in the third instance, the other parent was rated 3 (highly probable) for multiple personality disorder.

The contributions of Dr. Coons in Chapter 7 and Dr. Kluft in Chapters 8 and 9 also describe the cross-generational occurrence of multiple personality disorder. In a study of 20 multiple personality disorder patients, using a matched control group of 20 nonmultiple personality disorder, nonschizophrenic psychiatric patient controls, Dr. Coons found a very high rate of psychiatric disturbance (39 percent) among the children of the multiple personality disorder patients, compared with a 3.6 percent rate among children of the controls. One of the nine psychiatrically disturbed children of the multiple personality disorder patients, a 15-year-old boy who had been sexually abused by his father, had multiple personality disorder. Another of these nine, a four-year-old boy who was a sleepwalker, was diagnosed as having an atypical dissociative disorder.

Unfortunately, it is difficult to know the precise significance of his inclusion in such a vague classification. Two of the psychiatrically disturbed children of multiple personality disorder patients had disorders of physical rather than psychogenic origin. One, an incest child, had severe mental retardation. The other had mixed learning disabilities and impaired fine and gross motor control (probably secondary to malnutrition). The remaining five disturbed children of the multiple personality disorder patients had either established personality disorders (the two children over 18 years) or conduct disorders (three children ages nine to 17 years). From this small sample, it would seem that psychiatrically disturbed children of multiple personality disorder parents who develop psychogenic conditions will be most likely to have character pathology, a dissociative disorder, or both.

As Dr. Coons' group is followed, it will be of interest to see what further diagnoses may be made in their adult years. It will be important for these questions to be studied in larger samples. Given the fact that eight of the nine psychiatrically disturbed children of the multiple personality disorder patients were male, I am in full agreement with Dr. Coons' impression that they may have been the objects of "subtle retaliatory abuses" by their previously abused multiple personality disorder mothers. Just as Dr. Coons, I have also had a pregnant female multiple personality disorder patient whose hatred of men was translated into fantasies of abusing and mutilating her child if it were a boy. She wished for and had a girl, toward whom she has had a very loving and protective attitude.

In Chapter 8, Dr. Kluft notes the paucity of diagnosed children with multiple personality disorder (apparently only seven published cases of confirmed childhood multiple personality disorder, all since 1979) despite the very early first report of childhood multiple personality disorder by Despine in 1840. That case, however, was not known to most workers in the field. The major reasons for our failure to diagnose childhood multiple personality disorder relate to our general lack of awareness of the prevalence of multiple personality disorder and how to identify it, even in adults, and to the fact that most of those who have developed a serious interest in multiple personality disorder have tended to be in adult psychiatry.

It is evident from the experiences of Kluft and Fagan and McMahon (3) in treating even a small number of children that childhood is the optimal time to make the diagnosis and to intervene clinically. There is no comparison between the very brief, uncomplicated, relatively inexpensive and highly successful psychotherapy of childhood multiple personality disorder and the sometimes extremely long, difficult, highly complicated, extremely expensive, and often successful (but sometimes not) treatment of adulthood multiple personality disorder. A comparison of the treatment of "Bobby" with that of his mother makes this point. Intervention in childhood is also preventive: 1) of the further reinforcement and structuring of the dissociative defensive organization into the adult form of multiple personality disorder; 2) of many years of impaired functioning and often intense suffering; 3) of years of misdiagnosis and costly ineffectual treatment; 4) of long, arduous, painful, extremely costly treatment if the patient is correctly diagnosed in adulthood; 5) of a possible 39 percent rate of psychiatric disturbance in the multiple personality disorder child's children; and 6) of the transgenerational occurrence of multiple personality disorder and other dissociative disorders. Serious efforts at case-finding and accurate diagnosis would be a great bargain for everyone.

Kluft made a point of noting that case example 2 was referred as a case of childhood psychosis. From his brief description of the other four cases, it seems very likely that had case examples 1, 3, or 4 come to the attention of the mental health system under different circumstances (that is, to the attention of someone unfamiliar with multiple personality disorder), they might also have been diagnosed as psychotic.

We are only beginning to recognize that adult multiple personality disorder is much less rare than we believed it to be just a few years ago. We now have reason to be very seriously concerned about what has been and is happening to undiagnosed and misdiagnosed children with multiple personality disorder. There is much in this chapter that one might comment on, but I think it best to say that it is a chapter the reader should study thoroughly with regard to the similarities and differences between adult and childhood multiple personality disorder.

The same may be said of Dr. Kluft's Chapter 9, in which the major thrust is, in the author's own words in a separate communication, " . . . that unless we know what multiple personality disorder looks like when it does not look like classic multiple personality disorder, we will never appreciate the full nature of multiple personality disorder; and that childhood cases, and their differences from adult cases, are crucial to this." In this chapter, we are introduced to signs that should alert us to suspect the presence of multiple personality disorder. Kluft also describes forms of multiple personality disorder, latent and covert forms, that do not necessarily fulfill all DSM-III criteria, especially the third criterion of complexity, integration, and " . . . unique behavior patterns and social relationships" (at least as these requirements are currently understood), but which are here appropriately considered to be forms of multiple personality disorder.

CLOSING THOUGHTS

Whatever difficulties we may have as professionals in recognizing the existence of multiple personality disorder, there is no one who has greater difficulty believing it exists than the patients who have it. It is their defensive system, and, until treatment, their means of at least partially avoiding intense emotional pain. It is not uncommon for multiple personality disorder patients to pay "lip service" to their diagnosis for long periods of time before a true recognition and acceptance of their multiplicity is possible or tolerable.

Multiple personality disorder is a terrible illness to have. At best, it is a means of survival, of existing despite what Shengold has termed "soul murder" (4). At worst, it is a severely incapacitating, painful, bewildering, and persistent condition, that although treatable, is most often misdiagnosed for years, compounding the patient's suffering. If accurately diagnosed in adulthood, the treatment process may be long and extremely painful.

The chapters presented here indicate a pressing need for a markedly increased awareness among mental health professionals of the tragic frequency of child abuse and of the incidence of multiple personality disorder in both adults and children, which is much higher than previously appreciated. The term "mental health professionals" is used here in the broadest sense of its meaning: to include all possible case-finders, from school teachers and counselors to clergy, family physicians, pediatricians, social workers, and adult and child psychologists and psychiatrists.

It is imperative that training programs in these fields prepare their trainees to recognize and respond appropriately to these problems. In medical education, and particularly in psychiatric training, the curriculum must include adequate attention to the diagnosis and treatment of multiple personality disorder and other dissociative disorders. At present, few adult and even fewer child psychiatry residents receive anything close to sufficient instruction or supervision concerning these illnesses. Little is taught of their psychodynamics, their etiology, the historical data which it is necessary to collect in their assessment, the characteristic signs and symptoms, the interview techniques useful in eliciting them, or of the potentially effective treatment methods available for work with both adults and children. The first necessary step is to create an awareness that multiple personality disorder does, in fact, occur with a frequency that makes it likely that all psychiatric clinicians can expect to make the diagnosis, and that questions aimed at eliciting data concerning dissociative symptomatology, traumatization, and especially the various forms of child abuse, should be a routine part of the psychiatric history. Likewise, it is essential that currently practicing adult and child psychiatrists learn how to elicit and identify evidence of dissociative defenses during the mental status examination.

We are not yet able to state the dimensions of the problem of multiple personality disorder, but it may be, as some now suspect, that despite our advances, we are still seeing only the tip of a fairly large iceberg. In any event, it would appear that there is an opportunity at hand to learn a great deal, not so much about man's inhumanity to man in the abstract, as about his inhumanity to his own children. Perhaps, in the process, we can effect some change for the better, at least in the lives of those who seek our professional expertise.

References

1. Sandler J, Joffe WG: Towards a basic psychoanalytic model. Int J Psychoanal 50:79-90, 1969

2. Kluft RP: Treatment of multiple personality disorder: a study of 33 cases. Psychiatr Clin North Am 7:9-29, 1984

3. Fagan J, McMahon P: Incipient multiple personality in children: four cases. J Nerv Ment Dis 172:26-36, 1984

4. Shengold L: Child abuse and deprivation: soul murder. J Am Psychoanal Assoc 27:533-559, 1979